101 TIPS
for CHRONIC
PAIN RELIEF

Traditional, Alternative, and Complementary Health Solutions You can Use!

ALAN E. SMITH

Loving Healing Press

Ann Arbor, MI

ISBN 978-1-61599-851-7   paperback
ISBN 978-1-61599-852-4   hardcover
ISBN 978-1-61599-853-1   eBook

Published by
Loving Healing Press   info@LHPress.com
5145 Pontiac Trail   www.LHPress.com
Ann Arbor, MI 48105   Tollfree 888-761-6268
Distributed by Ingram Book Group (USA, CAN, EU, AU)

Library of Congress Cataloging-in-Publication Data
Names: Smith, Alan E., 1951- author.
Title: 101 tips for chronic pain relief : traditional, alternative, and
  complementary health solutions you can use! / Alan E. Smith.
Other titles: One hundred one tips for chronic pain relief
Description: Ann Arbor, MI : Loving Healing Press, [2025] | Includes
index.
  | Summary: "The author explores traditional, alternative, and
  complementary health solutions for chronic pain. Categories include
  electronic devices, over-the-counter drugs, prescriptions, mental
  therapies, and medical interventions. Complementary solutions such
  as pilates, yoga, massage, aromatherapy, and dozens of others are
  included"-- Provided by publisher.
Identifiers: LCCN 2024043974 (print) | LCCN 2024043975 (ebook) |
ISBN
  9781615998517 (paperback) | ISBN 9781615998524 (hardcover) |
ISBN
  9781615998531 (epub)
Subjects: LCSH: Chronic pain--Popular works. | Chronic
  pain--Treatment--Popular works.
Classification: LCC RB127 .S625 2025 (print) | LCC RB127 (ebook) |
DDC
  616/.0472--dc23/eng/20250124
LC record available at https://lccn.loc.gov/2024043974
LC ebook record available at https://lccn.loc.gov/2024043975

Contents

Why I Wrote This Book 1

Disclaimer 1

What You Need to Know About Pain.. 2

Devices to Relieve Your Pain 7

Tip #1: Virtual Reality (VR) Therapy 7

Tip #2: Biofeedback 7

Tip #3: Millimeter Wave Therapy 9

Tip #4: Infrared Therapy 9

Tip #5: Cold Laser 10

Tip #6: Green Light Therapy 11

Tip #7: Pulsetto 11

Tip #8: Cryotherapy.. 12

Tip #9: Percutaneous Electrical Nerve Stimulation (PENS) also Percutaneous Neuromodulation Therapy (PNT) 13

Tip #10: TENS (Transcutaneous Electrical Nerve Stimulator) 13

Tip #11: Smart Bandages... 14

Tip #12: High Frequency Impulse Therapy (HFIT)............... 14

Tip #13: Traction 15

Tip #14: Compression 16

Tip #15: Hydrotherapy 16

Over-The-Counter Pain Relief... 19

Tip #16: Aspirin 19

Tip #17: Alcohol 20

Tip #18: Hempvana™ 20

Tip #19: Biofreeze 21

Tip #20: Salonpas Pain Patch 21

Tip #21: Tylenol / Paracetamol..................................... 22

Tip #22: Advil 22

Tip #23: Emu Oil 23

Tip #24: Aspercreme 24

Tip #25: Heat & Cold 25

Tip #26: Arnicare 26

Tip #27: Omega XL 27

Tip #28: Icy Hot® 27

Tip #29: Tumeric (also Turmeric) 28

Tip #30: Thunder God Vine 28

Tip #31: Glucosamine and Chondroitin 29

Tip #32: Fish Oil 30

Tip #33: Gamma-linolenic Acid (GLA) 30

Tip #34: Capsaicin HP 30

Tip #35: Kratom 31

Tip #36: Voltaren 32

Prescribed Solutions 33

Tip #37: Vicodin 33

Tip #38: Fentanyl 33

Tip #39: Physical Therapy 34

Tip #40: Stem Cell Injection 35

Tip #41: Placebo 36

Tip #42: Injections 38

Tip #43: Tramadol 38

Tip #44: Medical Marijuana or Cannabis 39

Tip #45: Oxycodone 40

Tip #46: Percocet 41

Tip #47: Ubrelvy 42

Thinking About It 43

Tip #48: Humor Therapy 43

Tip #49: Hypnosis 44

Tip #50: Prayer Therapy.. 45

Tip #51: EFT or Emotional Freedom Technique.................... 46

Tip #52: PSYCH-K® 47

Tip #53: Mindfulness Based Stress Reduction 48

Tip #54: Mindfulness 49

Tip #55: Meditation 51

Tip #56: EMDR (Eye Movement Desensitization and
Reprocessing) 52

Tip #57: Cognitive-Behavioral Therapy (CBT) 53

Medical Solutions 55

Tip #58: Acupuncture.. 55

Tip #59: Osteopathic Medicine 56

Tip #60: Homeopathy 57

Tip #61: Ayurveda 59

Tip #62: Qi Gong or QiGong.. 60

Tip #63: Chiropractic.. 62

Tip #64: Surgical Intervention 63

Tip #65: S.C.E.N.A.R or SKENAR 64

Tip #66: Nerve Blocks 65

Tip #67: Implanted Spinal Cord Stimulation 66

Complementary and Alternative Medicine 67

Tip #68: Sound Therapy.. 67

Tip #69: Deep Oscillation 68

Tip #70: Pulsed Electro Magnetic Field (PEMF).................. 68

Tip #71: H-Wave.. 69

Tip #72: Feldenkrais Method®.. 69

Tip #73: Pilates 71

Tip #74: Applied Kinesiology 72

Tip #75: Healing Touch.. 73

Tip #76: Hellerwork Structural Integration 74

Tip #77: Bonnie Prudden Myotherapy 75

Tip #78: Rolfing Structural Integration 76

Tip #79: Massage 77

Tip #80: Yoga 79

Tip #81: The Alexander Technique 82

Tip #82: Naprapathy.. 84

Tip #83: Breathwork 85

Tip #84: Craniosacral Therapy 85

Tip #85: Magnetic Therapy 87

Tip #86: Reiki 88

Tip #87: Advanced Jaffe-Mellor Technique™ (JMT)......... 90

Tip #88: Energy Medicine 91

Tip #89: Bach Flower Therapy 92

Tip #90: Aromatherapy 94

Tip #91: Crystal Therapy 96

Tip #92: Water Therapy 98

Tip #93: Bee Venom Therapy 100

Tip #94: Art Therapy... 101

Tip #95: Music Therapy 101

Tip #96: Reflexology 102

Tip #97: Tai Chi 104

Tip #98: Quantum Techniques 105

Tip #99: Asian Bodywork... 106

Tip #100: Myofascial Release...................................... 107

Tip #101: The Yuen Method 108

Tip #102: Ozone or Oxygen Therapy........................... 109

The Message 110

About The Author... 113

Index.. 117

Why I Wrote This Book

I've watched chronic pain slowly eat away at a life. Sixty years ago, my mother was one of the first people in America to have a new surgical procedure developed in Europe to relieve pain in her spine. They took slivers of her hip bone and inserted them into her neck to separate the vertebrae and take pressure off the pinched nerves. It didn't work. It took nearly ten more years for her pain to finally end her life shortly after her fortieth birthday.

There have been many changes and improvements in pain treatment since then and I hope this book on 101 Tips for Chronic Pain will help you find some relief.

Disclaimer

This book is not intended to diagnose or prescribe any treatment for any medical or psychological condition(s), nor does it claim to prevent, diagnose, treat, mitigate, or cure any medical or psychological conditions.

It contains the ideas and opinions of its author and is intended solely to provide helpful information on a variety of subjects. It is sold with the understanding that the author and publisher are not engaged in rendering medical, health or any other kind of personal professional services in the book.

The reader should consult his or her medical, health or other competent professional before adopting any of the suggestions in the book.

The author and publisher specifically disclaim all responsibility for any liability, loss, or risk, personal or otherwise, that is incurred as a consequence (directly or indirectly) of the use and application of any of the contents of this book.

What You Need to Know About Pain

Pain. It can be low, pounding, never-seems-to-go-away pain or stabbing, piercing, want-to-scream-at-the-top-of-my-lungs pain. There are as many ways to describe pain as there are adjectives and adverbs in the English language. If you suffer from pain of any flavor, you want it to end as quickly as possible, and that's why you're reading this book.

What is pain? You know what it is: it's your nervous system telling you that something isn't right and it hurts. Pain is a complex process and it can vary from one person to the next even if they have similar injuries or illnesses. It begins with specialized nerve endings that are in almost all of your body tissues being activated after feeling pressure, temperature, irritation or simply to alert you to damage. Then the messages created by a stimulus are sent through specific nerves to the spinal cord where a filtering process can amplify or reduce the strength of the signal. Once in the spinal cord, different nerve cells relay the messages through well-defined pathways to higher processing centers in the brain such as the thalamus and cortex. Then you know it hurts. In other words, pain is a four-step process from transduction through transmission, modulation and eventually perception and it all happens incredibly fast.

Sometimes the signal outlasts its usefulness, hanging around after the original source of pain has been resolved or healed, and that's a challenge for modern medicine. Many people suffering with pain are told their pain is all in their head, which in a way it is. But advanced brain imaging has shown that those with chronic pain have clear differences in their brain activity.

There is acute pain and then there is chronic pain. A study in 2016 determined that about 20% of adults in America have chronic pain. Of those, about 8% suffer from what's called "high impact" chronic pain, which means pain that limits at least one major activity in their life. Chronic pain causes an estimated $560 billion every year in direct medical costs, lost productivity and disability programs in the USA. It's interesting that chronic pain seems to be a selective problem, occurring more frequently in women (about 70% of chronic pain patients), older adults, adults with public health insurance, rural residents, and those folks living in poverty. It happens less frequently among people with a bachelor's degree or higher. All in all, that's a lot of suffering. As common as chronic pain is, it doesn't even have a common definition, but you are the only one who knows what your pain feels like and that's all that matters.

It may be that poorly controlled acute pain leads to chronic pain, and stopping one will end the other, said Dr. Tina Doshi, a pain specialist at Johns Hopkins Medicine. But that's "hard to prove," she said.

The National Institute of Health (NIH) says: "Chronic pain is a medical disease that can be made worse by environmental and psychological factors. Chronic pain persists over a long period and can be challenging to manage. People with chronic pain often suffer from more than one painful condition. They also have an increased risk for developing problems with physical functioning, cognition, and emotional reactions. There may be common mechanisms that put some people at higher risk for developing multiple pain disorders. It is not known whether these disorders share a common cause."

According to the Mayo Clinic,

> Chronic pain is a serious health condition. Like any long-term health problem, it can lead to complications beyond physical symptoms such as depression, anxiety and trouble sleeping.

> Chronic pain is long-lasting. It can lead to problems with relationships and finances, makes it harder to keep up with work, tasks at home, and social gatherings. Some research suggests that the more severe the pain, the more serious these problems.

For these reasons, finding effective treatment for chronic pain is important, but the process is complex and personal. What works for one person's chronic lower back pain may not bring relief for another person's osteoarthritis.

There are a number of reasons for this. The cause of the chronic pain combined with a person's biology and history all play a role in pain management. Finding pain therapies that bring you relief can take time.

By working with your health care providers, you can find treatments that allow you to function better and live a more enjoyable, fulfilling life. The approach you choose should include more than medication. But medications may likely play a role.

The Cleveland Clinic's contribution is,

Chronic pain is pain that lasts for over three months. The pain can be there all the time, or it may come and go. It can happen anywhere in your body.

Chronic pain can interfere with your daily activities, such as working, having a social life and taking care of yourself or others. It can lead to depression, anxiety and trouble sleeping, which can make your pain worse. This response creates a cycle that's difficult to break.

Chronic pain differs from another type of pain called acute pain. Acute pain happens when you get hurt, such as experiencing a simple cut to your skin or a broken bone. It doesn't last long, and it goes away after your body heals from whatever caused the pain. In contrast, chronic pain continues long after you recover from an injury or illness. Sometimes it even happens for no obvious reason.

The folks at Johns Hopkins tell us,

Chronic pain is long standing pain that persists beyond the usual recovery period or occurs along with a chronic health condition, such as arthritis. Chronic pain may be "on" and "off" or continuous. It may affect people to the point that they can't work, eat properly, take part in physical activity, or enjoy life.

> Chronic pain is a major medical condition that can and should be treated.

> They add that chronic pain is defined as lasting more than three months.

The American Chronic Pain Association simply says that

> It's hard to know how to move forward once chronic pain has entered your life. It helps to think of a person with chronic pain like a car with four flat tires." It will take more than one type of therapy or treatment to get the car (your life) moving again.

> The National Center for Complementary and Integrative Health (a division of NIH) states that "Chronic pain is pain that lasts more than several months (variously defined as 3 to 6 months, but longer than "normal healing"). It's a very common problem.

Results from the 2019 National Health Interview Survey (NHIS) show that:

- About 20.4 percent of U.S adults had chronic pain (defined as pain on most days or every day in the past 3 months).

- About 7.4 percent of U.S. adults had high-impact chronic pain (defined as chronic pain that limited their life or work activities on most days or every day for the past 3 months).

It might be helpful at this point to add the most common 10-point Pain Rating Scale for future reference:

Rating	Subjective Description
0	…is no pain.
1 to 3	refers to mild pain.
4 to 6	refers to moderate pain.
7 to 10	refers to severe pain

While this book covers a wide variety of chronic pain treatments, I'd like to mention here that paying for many of the nondrug approaches can be challenging. Most insurance companies won't cover non-traditional treatments even though they have been proven effective.

Yes, we're talking about a lot of pain for a lot of people. Hopefully this collection of 101 Tips will help you find a way to treat your pain.

Devices to Relieve Your Pain

Tip #1: Virtual Reality (VR) Therapy

The pain of losing a limb has to be one of the worst type imaginable. Called Phantom Limb Pain, it's the result of an arm or leg being amputated. Afterward the patient may feel itching, burning, cramping or other sensations due to signals in the nervous system but without any way to relieve the pain, because the limb no longer exists. How can you scratch a leg that isn't there? Or put an ice pack on an arm that isn't there? The Cleveland Clinic estimates that 80% of amputees experience some type of phantom pain.

Current treatments include the traditional mirror therapy, prescription pain medications and even more surgery, but results with all of these are mixed. Today there is a new type of treatment being developed called Mixed Reality System for Managing Phantom Pain or Mr. MAPP. This high-tech version of the old mirror therapy gives patients a way for the brain to communicate with the missing limb. Using a virtual reality headset, the patient performs three exercises that require different motions, by playing games.

The system is still in development as they learn more about what works and what doesn't. One difference they've already discovered is that patients are more successful if they wear shorts with no shoes, for example, since they can "see" the real missing limb. This therapy convinces the brain that it's communicating with the missing limb, which relieves much of the pain and other sensations.

Tip #2: Biofeedback

Biofeedback is a process of recognizing the functioning of the body's systems in real time with the goal of correcting or improving performance. Change is accomplished by learning to modify the mind-body connection to alter muscle response, blood pressure and other bodily functions, including pain. The concept of voluntarily changing the autonomic nervous system through feedback was first studied in 1961.

Many people are familiar with the high-tech equipment often used in movies and sports to improve muscle tone and coordination, but a mirror can also be a biofeedback device. When a person simply watches the reflection of each step, they're learning to modify the signals from their mind to their body to improve walking. Whether the feedback is done with visual images, sounds, or both, it is a process to focus attention to learn improved control.

There are non-invasive devices that will measure muscle tension and brain waves for biofeedback. The term also includes other processes such as:

Electromyography (EMG)—a specialized device measures muscle tension, often used as therapy for headaches, morning stiffness, and fibromyalgia.

Thermal—the measurement of skin temperature has been found beneficial for Raynaud's Disease and other conditions involving reduced blood flow. It's also used to treat migraines.

GSR—Galvanic Skin Response is a measurement of the skin's conductivity, usually connected with an audible signal that becomes higher when stressed and lower when relaxed.

HRV—Heart Rate Variability measures changes in heartbeat as a biofeedback tool.

Respiration Training—uses various technologies to train and control breathing.

Electroencephalography or **EEG** biofeedback, also known as **Neurofeedback**, measures brainwaves by sensors attached to the scalp and each ear. Brain frequency activity is presented so specific frequencies can be stimulated or reduced. The technique has been found beneficial for many problems including ADD, learning difficulties, depression, and chronic fatigue.

Tip #3: Millimeter Wave Therapy

Millimeter Wave therapy (MW) is a non-invasive treatment considered to be a type of energy medicine. The original technology was developed in the Soviet Union during the Cold War for military purposes. The therapy has been used effectively in Russia and Eastern Europe for more than three decades to treat a wide variety of health problems including pain, skin diseases, wound healing, certain cancers, and gastrointestinal and cardiovascular diseases.

A Millimeter Wave device normally delivers a low-intensity, millimeter-wavelength electromagnetic beam to the skin at selected points such as an acupuncture point or a painful joint. The beam is absorbed at a very shallow level by the skin. This is a form of microwave which is non-ionizing, and there is no perceptible heating when used on a small area at a sufficiently low intensity. The radiation ranges from frequencies 30–300 GHz with the three most common frequencies used being 42.2, 53.6, and 61.2 GHz. The wavelengths involved range from 10 to 1 mm. Treatment time varies from 10 to 60 minutes and the results last from a few hours to several days. The treatment is painless, with exceedingly rare and minor side effects, and the technology involved is relatively inexpensive.

Research on the treatment in other countries has demonstrated an undisputed pain-relieving effect along with other beneficial results including normalizing the immune system, balancing metabolism, and increasing circulation to name just a few. MW therapy was studied in Russia from 1993-2003 on more than 20,000 patients, with 96% positive results. It is recommended for use by the Medical Health Ministry of the Russian Federation.

Tip #4: Infrared Therapy

Infrared Therapy for pain relief and control goes back to the 19th century, when we began to take advantage of this invisible electro-magnetic radiation. It is actually an extension of ancient healing techniques that used the power of the sun. This is not heat therapy, but light (or near light) therapy.

Many different devices are available for this type of therapy ranging from small, hand-held gadgets to lamps, to entire saunas. Infrared light enhances cell regeneration by producing nitric oxide that improves blood circulation, which brings more oxygen and nutrients to each cell. This also stimulates the mitochondria in your cells to produce more energy, especially in nerve cells. This regeneration of injured tissues reduces inflammation and pain.

A study in 2006 by the Rothbart Pain Management Clinic in Ontario, Canada, showed that chronic back pain could be reduced by up to 50% with Infrared Light Therapy, so keep this cheap alternative in your bag of chronic pain-relieving tricks.

Tip #5: Cold Laser

Cold lasers emit their photon energy with limited power that gently penetrates up to two inches below the surface of the skin with no tissue damage. Technically speaking, this amounts a few Joules per square-centimeter (J / cm^2) with laser power of 50 milliwatts (mW) or less. There is no heat or pain from this type of device and it is being used to treat a variety of health problems including chronic pain.

The Food & Drug Administration (FDA) first approved the use of cold laser therapy to treat neck and shoulder pain, following with approval for carpal tunnel syndrome in 2002, but most insurance companies deny coverage, considering the technology experimental. A variety of devices is used to treat a range of inflamed conditions of soft tissues and joints such as sports injuries, arthritis, back pain, and other injuries to the musculoskeletal system. Cold lasers are even being used as "pointless" acupuncture, with light energy stimulating the acupuncture points without pain and improving lymph drainage.

One type of device is Anodyne® Therapy, which comes from the word anodyne, meaning a medical treatment that soothes or relieves pain. This device uses monochromatic near-infrared photo energy (MIRE) with pads that emit the light applied to the surface of the skin. The technique usually focuses on the feet, often those with diabetes or PAD. It was approved by the FDA and first used in 1994.

Tip #6: Green Light Therapy

Why in the world would a different color of light reduce and even eliminate chronic pain? Today there are a lot of scientists all over the world asking and researching that same question. Recent interest is trying to discover the answer to questions like why different shades of green affect different people differently, and how it impacts pain in the first place. The bottom line is that green light can reduce the frequency and severity of pain from chronic muscle and skeletal pain as well as migraines, fibromyalgia, and other issues.

Modern research was ignited by Mahob M. Ibrahim, director of the Chronic Pain Management Clinic at the University of Arizona College of Medicine. His brother had told him that just sitting among the trees in his backyard would reduce his headaches. When Dr. Ibrahim started getting a headache he began walking in the greenery in a park and he also felt better, which got him started on answering the question of why. The mechanism involved in this pain modulation isn't yet understood, but green light appears to interrupt the pain connection in the brain. Right now, we don't even know which colors or intensities of green make the difference in particular types of pain. There aren't even any guidelines on the treatment duration. If walking in the forest isn't an option, there are many different types of devices from glasses to lightboxes and bulbs that you can experiment with to find your own therapy.

Tip #7: Pulsetto

The Pulsetto is a wearable device to stimulate the vagus nerve, the main pathway for the parasympathetic nervous system, which interacts with the parts of the brain responsible for processing pain signals. It's similar to other devices like the GammaCore, Nurosym, Sensate, Vagustim, Sapphire, taVNS and others. This vagus nerve stimulation or VNS device is used to treat chronic pain syndrome,

Parkinson's disease, epilepsy, cerebral palsy and other health problems. It has been used since the 1990s to treat chronic cluster headaches and to reduce chronic pain.

The first thing to do is lubricate your neck with the enclosed gel, similar to what's used for an ultrasound, to provide better electrical contact, and then put it around your neck. The device is then connected to a phone app, which offers five stimulation programs, one of which is specifically designed for pain, and nine stimulation frequency levels. Treatments range from four to 20 minutes.

The Pulsetto must fit around your neck correctly to stimulate the vagus nerve. While it works for most people, there are reports of smaller women finding the neckband too large for their neck. Be warned that folks with certain health conditions such as heart issues, epilepsy, or those with an implanted device should exercise extreme caution and check with their doctor before using.

Tip #8: Cryotherapy

Remember when you were a kid and dropped something on your toe and your Mom put an ice pack or a bag of ice cubes or even a bag of frozen peas on it to make it feel better? Cryotherapy, also known as cold therapy, uses low temperatures to treat pain and reduce inflammation. The human body releases endorphins when it's exposed to cold temperatures. Endorphins are hormones that act as powerful natural painkillers.

Today there are many improvements to Mom's bag of ice cubes. Now we have machines you can buy or rent that circulate ice water through special pads so they can be used on any part of your body. Pain therapy specialists have even better cryogenic equipment to relieve your pain.

Cold therapy should only be used for short periods of time, usually up to 15 minutes, to prevent nerve or tissue damage and never on stiff muscles or joints. People with sensory disorders that reduce their ability to feel sensations should not use cold therapy at home, because they may not be able to feel if damage is being done.

For example, people with diabetes may have decreased sensitivity and should restrict any use of cold therapy.

Tip #9: Percutaneous Electrical Nerve Stimulation (PENS) also Percutaneous Neuromodulation Therapy (PNT)

A single event of back pain can cause the nerve cells to become hypersensitive, a chronic pain condition that can continue long after the original injury. Percutaneous Electrical Nerve Stimulation (PENS) and Percutaneous Neuromodulation Therapy (PNT) are both low-risk therapies relying on inserting fine needles through the skin, similar to electrical acupuncture, but placement is not determined by energy meridians as it is with Traditional Chinese Medicine.

Both PENS and PNT are based on inserting fine-gauge electrodes (about 250 microns in diameter) to a depth of 1 to 4 cm with electrical stimulation of 15 to 30 Hz. Placement is guided by the location of the pain. By comparison, PNT therapy places up to 10 electrodes at specific locations in the back. Treatment protocols are for 30-minute sessions up to three times per week for up to ten sessions. Both types of treatment devices have been approved by the FDA) for patients suffering from chronic low back or neck pain.

Tip #10: TENS (Transcutaneous Electrical Nerve Stimulator)

TENS or Transcutaneous Electrical Nerve Stimulator, is a pocket-sized electronic device that generates electrical signals to stimulate nerves through the skin for pain relief, frequently for the back. A typical unit is battery-powered with controls for frequency and intensity, a pulse generator, and a transformer. The unit is connected by wires to electrodes that stick on the skin.

The TENS unit controls pain by sending electrical signals to the nerves blocking the pain signal to the brain. The positioning of the electrodes on the skin determines which muscles and nerves are stimulated. TENS may also work by stimulating the body's own endorphins in the brain, which act to reduce pain.

Electrical stimulation for pain control actually goes back to ancient Greece. Early devices were developed back in the 16th century. The modern, wearable TENS was patented in 1974 and was originally used for testing patient tolerance to electrical stimulation before a device was implanted in their spinal cord. Many of the patients got so much relief from the TENS unit that they never had the surgery.

Tip #11: Smart Bandages

For those of you who suffer from a wound or injury that just won't heal, you already know how painful it can be. Chronic non-healing wounds are a major medical challenge that can lead to eventual amputation. There is hope on the horizon though in the form a "smart bandage," which can sense and respond to a variety of issues with a wound.

Testing with mice has already produced bandages that can reduce infection and even accelerate wound healing. These wirelessly powered, closed-loop sensing and stimulation bandages have already produced an improvement in healing time of 25% with better skin repair.

Basically, a bandage can have sensors to monitor wound temperature, oxygen saturation, pH (acidity), electrical conductivity, and wound pressure activity to monitor temperature changes, oxygen/moisture content and other factors. This information can be stored or transmitted to a remote device for your doctor's review.

Tip #12: High Frequency Impulse Therapy (HFIT)

If you have chronic low-back pain, this one may be of particular interest to you. This is a device you wear that delivers electric impulses like a TENS unit but with high-frequency components. This combination produces a nerve-block effect, which reduces pain. The ultra-high frequency system involves waveforms in the 30-150 kHz range to overcome skin resistance and deliver a higher frequency than a TENS unit. In a double-blind clinical trial, it was able to reduce pain by 56% for up to 86% of patients. You shouldn't use HFIT if you're pregnant, have severe epilepsy or have any electronic implant.

Tip #13: Traction

If your chronic pain comes from your lower back or your neck or anything in between, this should be of particular interest to you. Traction is called non-surgical spinal decompression, and a wide variety of devices is available to provide traction ranging from the neck and shoulders down to the waist. It can be delivered horizontally, vertically and even inverted. Be sure to talk with your doctor before using any at-home traction device.

Traction is a way to relieve painful pressure on/in the spine. It's used to treat everything from low back and neck pain to weakness, numbness, or electrical sensations going down your arm or leg. It can be done manually by a physical therapist or mechanically either with your therapist or at home. Spinal traction is used to treat herniated or slipped discs, sciatica, degenerative disc disease, pinched nerves in the spine, and many other issues.

A 2022 study found lumbar traction beneficial for people with low back pain and that high-force lumbar traction was able to reduce functional disability. However, be aware that spinal traction can sometimes cause pain that is actually worse than the original condition. It can also cause muscle spasms. People with osteoporosis and certain types of cancer should not use traction therapy.

I have to add that my personal favorite in this category is a back decompression belt lumbar support waist air traction brace. As we know it takes very little motion to relieve pressure and pain on the spine and this at-home device is just what I need when my lower back is unhappy. For the record, there are even videos on a wide range of traction devices available on YouTube.com.

Tip #14: Compression

Sometimes there are things you can do outside your body that can help with your pain or to even prevent pain. Compression is one of those steps you can take on your own. Compression therapy increases blood circulation and reduces pain with a variety of wearable devices ranging from socks (long and short) to knees to lower back to hands and wrists even to an eye mask for headache pain.

Compression therapy helps increase blood circulation and it's especially effective in the lower legs, ankles and feet. It is an effective treatment for pain and swelling caused by conditions associated with poor circulation, so whether you're on your feet all day or sitting at a desk, compression socks can help with your pain and circulation. They can also be worn on long airline flights to prevent Deep Vein Thrombosis (DVT). Whether you stand up all day at work or sit at a desk all day, compression stockings can be a big help in keeping you pain-free and comfortable. Compression therapy can also help people suffering from fibromyalgia and lymphatic diseases, arthritis and those with venous ulcers and swelling.

Some athletes involved in endurance sports use compression therapy on their legs either during or after exercise. The increased blood circulation is thought to improve muscle recovery and reduce soreness.

A wide variety of devices ranging from bandages to intermittent pneumatic compression (IPC) systems use cuffs around the legs. You can buy many of these devices over-the-counter or at a medical supply store. There are even devices that offer additional benefits in addition to compression, like Copper Fit gloves and braces. The key for any type of compression device is to find the correct size for you and learn how best to wear it.

Tip #15: Hydrotherapy

Hydrotherapy is using water for health, and hydrothermal therapy adds temperature, as in hot baths or saunas. This is one of the oldest forms of therapy going back to ancient Greeks. Public communal baths were also part of ancient Rome. China and Japan also had bathing as part of their ancient cultures. Being immersed or doing exercises in water has been a popular therapy in many cultures for thousands of years.

There are many different methods of hydrotherapy including: baths and showers; colonics; douches; localized therapies like sitz or foot baths; steam inhalation; hot compresses, and body wraps, to name just a few. The healing properties of water are based on its mechanical effects (either pressure or jets) or its thermal effects. In addition, various herbs or salts may be used to enhance the experience. Heated water in a whirlpool or bath naturally soothes the body while the weightlessness of being in water helps to relieve stress and muscle tension and thereby easing pain. When pressurized jets are used, circulation is boosted, helping to release tight muscles. From spas in Europe to thermal springs across America like Hot Springs, Arkansas and Palm Springs, California, hot water therapy has always been popular. These naturally heated hot springs often contain a variety of minerals, which are promoted as having special healing powers.

A sauna, also called a Turkish or hot air bath, can have temperatures of 120 to 212 degrees, with 150 degrees Fahrenheit being the norm. There are also moist air steam baths. In either case, the heat stimulates the body to sweat toxins out through the skin. They also stimulate blood flow, increase heart rate, open airways and promote hormone production. Exposure can range from twenty minutes up to two hours. This is similar to the sweat lodge used by Native American Indian tribes.

Another common type of hydrotherapy is a wrap, either hot or cold. Primarily used as a supportive measure for treating fever and local inflammation, a moistened cloth is wrapped around the body or its affected part and then covered with a dry cloth. If a cool wrap is used to reduce inflammation, the process will probably last 45 minutes to an hour. If a warm cloth is used to produce sweating, the procedure may last hours.

When using a spa or hot tub, a neutral temperature ranging between 92 and 94 degrees is recommended to relieve tension, but a higher temperature of 102 to 106 degrees is often suggested if the goal is to relax muscles. Taking a cold shower after a hot bath can be very invigorating but be cautious because it can also be very dangerous.

Please consult your doctor to determine if this type of therapy is suitable for your condition. Many people should avoid it. People with diabetes should avoid any hot body wrap but especially to their feet or legs. Immersion in hot baths or using hot saunas is not recommended for diabetics, pregnant women, and people with multiple sclerosis or anyone with abnormally high or low blood pressure. The elderly and children should also exercise caution. Always be sure to drink plenty of water to replace what's been lost.

Over-The-Counter Pain Relief

Tip #16: Aspirin

Aspirin is one of the oldest medicines available for pain relief and it's the most widely used drug in the world today. Willow bark has been used as a medicine for thousands of years and salicin is its effective ingredient. Aspirin is a salicylate that works to reduce substances in the body that can cause pain, fever, and inflammation. It can even be used to prevent heart attacks, strokes and chest pain or to treat those conditions. It was synthesized by the folks at Bayer at the end of the 19th century. Today, aspirin is available from baby aspirins to coated aspirins to prescription aspirin which is used to relieve the pain of rheumatoid arthritis, osteoarthritis and other rheumatologic conditions.

It is often recommended to take aspirin with food to prevent it upsetting your stomach. The Mayo Clinic website lists over 60 side effects of aspirin. You shouldn't take aspirin if you have hemophilia or intestinal bleeding. Avoid aspirin if you are allergic to an NSAID (non-steroidal anti-inflammatory drug) such as Advil, Motrin, Aleve or other similar drug. Also avoid drinking while you're taking aspirin since it can increase your risk of stomach bleeding.

Never give aspirin to a child or teenager with a fever, flu symptoms or chickenpox. Taking aspirin late in a pregnancy may cause bleeding in the mother or baby during delivery. Aspirin can also pass into breast milk and harm a baby.

To make sure aspirin is safe, be sure to tell your doctor if you have asthma or seasonal allergies, stomach ulcers, liver or kidney disease, gout, heart disease or high blood pressure.

Tip #17: Alcohol

there has been alcohol almost since the beginning of human history, and sad to say, it seems to be a pretty effective pain reliever. Science doesn't know why it works, only that it works, so well that an estimated 28% of chronic pain sufferers turn to alcohol for their symptoms. Not that scientists haven't tried to figure out why it's even better than some painkillers, in fact recent research examined 18 different studies on pain showing how effective it is.

Many drinkers turned to alcohol for pain relief for its ability to depress the central nervous system, or in other words, pain relief. The issue is, how much and how often. It appears that after three drinks for men and two drinks for women, the painkilling effectiveness can be described as "moderate to large." Unfortunately, the Dietary Guidelines for Americans 2020-2025 recommend only two drinks per day for men and only one drink per day for women. However, booze is cheaper than most prescription drugs, which makes it very attractive. However, eventually you'll have to drink more and more to get the same amount of pain relief. That's how an alcoholic is created. Being in chronic pain leads to alcohol abuse, which is basically trading one problem for another.

Using alcohol and opioids together can cause an overdose because it depresses parts of the brain that control breathing. In fact, research seems to suggest that alcohol is involved in about one in five deaths from opioid overdoses. But the dangers of alcohol aren't just with opioids. If you've ever taken an over-the-counter pain reliever like Tylenol, Advil or Aleve after a night of drinking to treat your hangover, you may also be creating an ulcer, stomach bleeding, liver and kidney damage and more. Withdrawing from chronic alcohol use can not only increase pain sensitivity but it's frequently a motivation for some to increase their drinking.

Tip #18: Hempvana™

One of the newer over-the-counter (OTC) pain solutions is Hempvana, which is a pain relief cream with hemp seed oil. It relieves both pain and inflammation. One of its advantages is that it treats the pain and not the entire body like a drug. The key to its effectiveness is that it contains CBD from the oil of the seeds of the Cannabis Sativa plant, but it does not get you "high" because it does not contain THC, which is what causes psychotropic effects. This topical pain relief product is produced in America in an FDA-registered facility. Warnings on the jar say not to use more than three times each day.

Tip #19: Biofreeze

Biofreeze is the brand name of a menthol topical medicine that's been around for over 25 years. It's made from extracts of mint oil and provides a cooling sensation when applied to the skin. This feeling of cooling helps to relieve pain temporarily in the tissues underneath the skin, such as muscles. It's used to treat joint pain and even bruises, and is even been used for arthritis pain. The major ingredient is menthol, which stimulates the thermoreceptors in the skin, giving a cooling sensation, which then stimulates non-nociceptive nerve fibers that act as a counterirritant. It also causes vasodilation, which improves blood flow and improves lymphatic drainage, which also reduces inflammation.

This product is non-systemic, non-narcotic and contains no NSAIDs, salicylates or any addictive substance. It comes in a variety of products including gel, spray, roll-on, cream, in a large patch, single-use patches, pump, foam, pen and strip. Do not apply to serious burns or deep wounds. Do not use on broken or irritated skin and on open wounds. Do not cover the treated area with a heating pad or with a tight bandage. It should not be used more than three or four times per day. Rinse with water if it gets into your eyes or mouth. For your first use, only apply Biofreeze to a small area of skin to see how it reacts.

Tip #20: Salonpas Pain Patch

Salonpas Pain Patch (for the skin) is used for temporary relief of minor aches and pains caused by everything from strains and sprains to arthritis, bruising, nerve pain, down to a simple backache. There are different types of patches available over the counter, depending on your pain and its location. One type of patch contains a 4% Lidocaine ingredient while another uses a combination of 3% Menthol and 10% Menthyl Salicylate. In addition to patches, Salonpas also offers gels and even spray products for pain relief. Please note that you should never cover treated skin with a bandage or heating pad.

Tip #21: Tylenol / Paracetamol

Tylenol™, or acetaminophen, is an over-the-counter pain reliever for a wide variety of pain ranging from headaches and arthritic pain to all types of muscle and even sinus pain. It's available in tablets, capsules, liquid, chewable tablets and dissolvable powders. Outside North America, acetaminophen is branded as Panadol™ or generically as Paracetamol. Rest assured that all four of these names are chemically identical to each other: Tylenol, acetaminophen, Panadol, and Paracetamol. This is an important fact for world travelers to know!

Be warned that anyone weighing at least 110 pounds should not take more than 1000 milligrams at one time or more than 4000 mg in 24 hours. If you drink more than three drinks per, day you may not be able to take Tylenol because it can damage your liver. Stop taking Tylenol and contact your doctor if you continue to have a sore throat after using it for two days, or if you still have a fever after three days. Obviously, call your doctor immediately if you develop a skin rash or nausea, vomiting, swelling or other serious reaction. While this may be an over-the-counter medication, it is still potentially dangerous.

Tip #22: Advil

Advil, or ibuprofen, which is its generic name, is a nonsteroidal anti-inflammatory drug that eases pain by reducing certain hormones in the body. By lowering inflammation, it reduces your pain, fever and other issues, which is why it's recommended for everything from headache to a toothache.

There are several variations of Advil but normally the product is taken by mouth every four to six hours with a full glass of water. Don't take any more of it or take it any more frequently than recommended, as it can damage your stomach and intestines. It's usually recommended that you take it with food or milk. Also, do not lie down for at least ten minutes after taking an Advil.

There can be adverse reactions as with any over-the-counter medication. Advil can increase the risk of a fatal heart attack or stroke, even if you don't have any of the normal risk factors. It can also cause stomach or intestinal bleeding, which can also be fatal, and these risks increase for elderly patients.

Tip #23: Emu Oil

Who would have thought we'd be talking about large, flightless birds originally from Australia? But the Aboriginal people there have reportedly used Emu oil for more than 40,000 years. When emus started being raised for their meat in America, it was only a matter of time before emu oil was used for pain relief.

There are many types of emu oil products available today, but Blue Emu cream is probably the best known. It contains glucosamine and methylsulfonylmethane (MSM) added to emu oil along with aloe vera. It's rich in essential fatty acids—omega 3, 6, and 9. Oleic acid (a monounsaturated omega-9 fatty acid). Emu oil is a natural type of transdermal carrier, which simply means it can penetrate the skin with its anti-inflammatory, antibacterial and anti-fungal properties.

A study reported in the National Library of Medicine says that Emu oil has been found to help relieve muscle pain and treat inflamed joints. This makes it perfect for back pain, painful joints and for arthritic pain.

It's very simply to use Emu oil products. Simply rub a thin layer on the painful area. Although it is not recommended to put it on cuts, open wounds or any type of damaged skin, Australian aborigines find it to be soothing and to alleviate scar tissue. Don't wrap the area too tightly with a bandage or use any type of heating pad or other heating device.

While it's rare, some people may have very bad and sometimes deadly side effects. Get medical help immediately if you show any signs of an allergic reaction like a rash, hives or any type of skin reaction. This could lead to fever, trouble breathing or swallowing and swelling of the mouth, lips, tongue or throat.

Tip #24: Aspercreme

Aspercreme is an over-the-counter (OTC) treatment for all types of pain ranging from strains and sprains to back aches to arthritis and almost everything in between. The original product contains trolamine salicylate as its active ingredient but today it comes in a variety of forms with additional active ingredients such as lidocaine HCl or diclofenac topical gel. One of the major advantages of this product is that it can be placed directly on the source of pain in your body.

It's recommended that you don't use it more than three or four times per day. If you're using a form of Aspercreme with diclofenac topical gel, don't apply more than 16 grams to any single joint of the lower body such as your knee or ankle. Don't use more than 8 grams to any single part of the upper body like your wrist or elbow. Whatever you're treating, don't use more than 32 grams of diclofenac in a single day. Always avoid getting it in your mucous membranes like the lining of your nose. Never apply it to any area of the skin that's already irritated or damaged. Don't use it over large areas of the body. After you apply it, don't wrap a bandage too tightly so the area can't breathe properly and never put a heating pad on Aspercreme. After rubbing it on, you should always remember to wash your hands thoroughly. Be aware that if you're treating your arthritis it may take up to two weeks to get the full benefit.

Tip #25: Heat & Cold

These are some of the oldest pain treatments known. We've already discussed cold therapy, also known as **Cryotherapy**, earlier. I'll just add here that cold therapy always needs to be used for a limited amount of time per session. Because it's best used to reduce inflammation and acute pain, you should always have an ice pack in the freezer or at least a bag of frozen vegetables (peas work best).

A recent survey by the U.S. Pain Foundation found heat and cold therapies are the most common relief options for people with chronic pain. The survey showed that almost 68% said they use heat at least once each week while almost 45% said they use cold therapy at least once per week. It was interesting that just over half of the folks responding to the survey said they found heat to be more effective while less than 20% preferred cold. About 29% said they were about equal.

Heat therapy helps to improve blood flow to the painful area, bringing additional nutrients so it's effective for muscle pain and stiffness. This means it's great to warm up muscles before an activity. Obviously you should never use heat therapy to an open wound. There are two types of heat therapy: dry heat and moist heat. Both aim to be really "warm" instead of hot. The advantage is you can choose to use heat therapy for a small part or large part of your body or even your entire body if you want to use a sauna or hot bath.

Dry heat, also called conducted heat therapy, uses a variety of tools from a hot water bottle (very old school) to heating pads that can be warmed up in the microwave, or pads that can simply be plugged in. Moist heat or convection heat uses steamed towels, moist heating packs and can even use a warm wax device for smaller parts of the body like hands and feet. There are also professional heat treatments that can be used including heat from an ultrasound. Since moist heat seems to be slightly more effective, it may require less time.

People with certain medical conditions shouldn't use heat therapy at all due to a higher risk of burns or complications. If you have diabetes, dermatitis, vascular diseases, deep vein thrombosis, or multiple sclerosis (MS), don't use heat therapy.

If you want to use both heat, and cold therapies apply heat for up to 20 minutes and then a few hours later you can use ice for up to 20 minutes. Using these spaced intervals, you can do this several times each day to reduce inflammation and loosen your muscles at the same time while increasing your pain relief.

Tip #26: Arnicare

Arnicare is a remedy that's been used for centuries so there must be something beneficial in it. It comes from the Arnica Montana plant, which is a perennial that grows one to two feet tall with bright yellow and orange daisy-like flowers. It's normally found in the Northwestern United States but also on the moist, grassy upland meadows in the hills and mountains of central Europe and Siberia. It's also called the mountain daisy, leopard's bane, and mountain tobacco.

St. Hildegard was a German nun in the 12th century known for her observations of nature, and she wrote about the healing properties of the Arnica Montana plant. It's been used by the mountain people since the 16th century to relieve muscle aches, pains and even bruises. Today it has grown into one of the most popular homeopathic medicines in the world. It's available as an ointment, gel or cream and when diluted homeopathically, it can be taken internally. However, it contains a toxin called helenalin, which can be deadly when consumed in large quantities. This is why several countries have banned its use in any culinary product.

It is an effective herbal therapy for a wide range of aches and pains, even osteoarthritis. A 2021 review of studies on herbal therapies found that arnica gel is about as effective as topical NSAIDS for inflammation and pain relief. There is even an Arnicare Arthritis formulation, which is perfect for those concerned about drug interactions and pre-existing conditions.

Arnicare shouldn't be used on children under 12 years of age. Avoid contact with your eyes, mucous membranes and damaged skin. All of the creams and ointments are for external use only. Never wrap a bandage too tightly after applying Arnicare or use heat or ice to treat the area immediately after application.

Tip #27: Omega XL

This is a supplement claiming to improve joint health, reduce inflammation and relieve pain associated with osteoarthritis and rheumatoid arthritis by using fatty acids including Omega-3. It is produced by Great Health Works from Green Lipped Mussels farmed in New Zealand and is supposed to be twenty times more powerful than standard fish oil. It does not contain shellfish allergens.

The Food & Drug Administration (FDA) has not approved Omega XL as a drug to prevent, treat or cure any disease. In 2021 they warned Great Health Works about medical claims made on their website about Omega XL.

The product is said to be backed more than 35 years of clinical research but the evidence is mixed on the question of whether it actually works. Research does indicate that improving your omega 3:6 ratio can improve your health but it also indicates that omega-3 supplements aren't as effective as simply eating seafood.

There can be side effects to Omega XL including gout, heartburn, nausea and diarrhea.

Omega XL's reviews on Amazon are mostly positive but the reviews for the company, Great Health Works, are not.

Tip #28: Icy Hot®

I'm sure you've seen the TV commercials for this pain-relief product. The name says it all: it delivers a two-step process that feels icy at first to dull the pain and then it feels hot to relax it. This is possible by using 16% menthol and 11% camphor together although they add additional ingredients like methyl salicylate or lidocaine in some of their products. It's available in patches, sleeves, balms, roll-ons, dry sprays, gels and creams. Pain relief can last up to 12 hours.

As I've said before with this type of over-the-counter product, never put it near your eyes, mouth, nose or genitals, and if you do, rinse it thoroughly with water. Never put it on any skin that is cut, scraped, sunburned or damaged in any way. Be sure to never cover the treated skin with a bandage or heating pad.

Tip #29: Tumeric (also Turmeric)

If you suffer from the chronic pain of arthritis this is an especially important listing for you. While the terms "turmeric" and "curcumin" are sometimes used interchangeably, they actually mean different things. Tumeric, also spelled Turmeric, comes from the root of the curcuma longa plant, a perennial in the ginger family, while curcumin is the compound found in turmeric that gives it that distinctive yellowish color. Turmeric is sometimes called the "golden spice," so confusion is common. It's also called Indian saffron, probably because India produces nearly all of the world's turmeric crop and consumes 80% of it.

Tumeric has been used in medicine for almost 4,000 years because of its antioxidant and anti-inflammatory properties. It has deep roots in both Traditional Chinese Medicine and traditional Ayurveda. Modern medicine is beginning to recognize its importance, showing up in over 3,000 publications in the past 25 years. A 2016 research review found that curcumin may relieve joint pain as effectively as NSAIDs in people with rheumatoid arthritis and osteoarthritis.

Don't confuse turmeric with Javanese turmeric root, tree turmeric, zedoary or goldenseal. Turmeric can lessen the effects of aspirin, ibuprofen and acetaminophen. It can also increase your risk of kidney stones.

Tip #30: Thunder God Vine

Thunder God Vine, also known as Lei Gong Teng in Chinese, is a woody plant that grows close to water sources in the mountainous regions of Southern China, Korea, Japan, and Taiwan. Its leaves and root have been used for many centuries as part of Traditional

Chinese Medicine. It is reported to have a unique ability to regulate the immune system and reduce inflammation, which is why it's used to treat the pain of rheumatoid arthritis (RA) and other auto-immune diseases.

The traditional use of Thunder God Vine is to skin the root of the vine and then reduce the extract into a powder that can then be taken with water. It can also be applied to the skin over the painful joints to decrease tenderness, stiffness and swelling. In studies it's been shown to be as effective as conventional drugs. It can also improve the effectiveness of non-steroidal anti-inflammatory drugs (NSAIDs) when taken with them. The active ingredient in Thunder God Vine is Triptolide.

Side effects can be dangerous including skin rashes, nausea, headaches and even loss of bone density, so you'll need to check with your physician and also with a trained herbalist. Unfortunately, it's reported that over 50% of Thunder God Vine products are adulterated with a cheaper plant called Kupiteng in Chinese.

Tip #31: Glucosamine and Chondroitin

I have to include these two because there are too many folks who swear by it. The reason there are two chemicals togethers is because you frequently see them together in products like Move Free and many others, but they can be bought separately. Chondroitin is believed to help you maintain fluid and flexibility in your joints. Meanwhile Glucosamine helps you build cartilage. Cartilage is a type of connective tissue that protects and cushions the bones.

People with osteoarthritis know that their cartilage has worn down and the bones are rubbing together in a painful manner. Since 3.6% of the population suffer with osteoarthritis, they're looking for this type of specific pain relief. The combination of Glucosamine and Chondroitin work together for just this reason. Many European countries actually prescribe them to relieve this type of pain. What's interesting is that the results of studies in the U.S. are mixed at best, with some showing no benefit at all. The good news is, these appear to be safe and may be helpful, which is especially important for those folks who can't take NSAIDs.

Tip #32: Fish Oil

Fish oil is one of the most popular types of over-the-counter (OTC) supplements. It may come from many types of fish but its effectiveness is from having two different types of omega-3 fatty acids called eicosapentaenoic acid (EPA) and docosahexaenoic acid (DHA). If you have Rheumatoid Arthritis, clinical trials have shown that it may help relieve tender joints and morning stiffness, enough so you can reduce the amount of NSAIDs you take every day. It may also relieve chronic inflammation.

Fish oil is generally considered to be safe with a dose of 3 grams or less each day. Taking more may increase the chance of bleeding. Side effects include heartburn, loose stools, nosebleeds and what are known as "fish burps" which is an unpleasant taste.

Tip #33: Gamma-linolenic Acid (GLA)

As long as I'm on the subject of fatty acids, let's add GLA to the list. It is found in oils from plants including evening primrose, borage, and black currant seed oils. This is a polyunsaturated fat, meaning it's a type of fat your body can't make, so normally we get GLA in 5% to 10% of the foods we eat.

As with Fish Oil, this is supposed to help relieve the pain and inflammation of rheumatoid arthritis,s and help with other autoimmune conditions. If you're going to use GLA for arthritis, realize that it can take one to three months to see any benefit and it's unlikely that it will stop the progression of the condition. GLA may also increase the risk of bleeding in folks taking anticoagulants and blood thinners.

Tip #34: Capsaicin HP

If you've ever had a bite of a fresh pepper and felt that burning, stinging sensation then you already know what Capsaicin is: it makes peppers hot. It can also be used to confuse your nervous system and hide the pain in your muscles and joints. Its medicinal use dates back 7,000 years in Mexico and it also has antimicrobial and anticancer properties.

Capsaicin is used in a variety of creams, gels, patches, ointments and lotions, interacts with nerve receptor TRPV1, and reduces the amount of substance P, a chemical that acts as a pain messenger in the body. It is beneficial for reducing pain in rheumatoid arthritis, osteoarthritis and even fibromyalgia. Use it only on the skin by applying a thin layer on the affected area and rubbing it in gently. Never apply this type of medication to the eyes, mouth, nostrils or genitals, but if it happens, flush the area with plenty of water. Also, do not apply to skin that is injured or irritated. Don't use it right before or after bathing, swimming, sunbathing or heavy exercise. Never wrap or bandage the affected area or use a heating pad.

If you suffer severe burning, pain, swelling or blistering of the skin, get emergency medical attention. Also watch for an allergic reaction such as hives, difficulty breathing, swelling of your face, lips, tongue or throat.

Tip #35: Kratom

Mitra Gyna speciosa or A. Kratom is an evergreen tree in the coffee family found in Southeast Asia and Africa. It produces an herbal extract called Kratom but it has a variety of street names like Thang, Krypton, Thom, Ketum, cratom, gratom, katawn and ithang. This extract is marketed as a treatment for muscle pain and it comes in a variety of forms from liquid to pills to powders and it can even be brewed. The safe dose of Kratom will vary .based on age, gender, weight, metabolism, diet and other factors.

It is believed to act on opioid receptors, and at relatively high doses can reduce pain and bring on a feeling of euphoria. Chronic use of opioid painkillers can lead to hyperalgesia, which is the upregulation of your pain sensitivity. This means if you use it daily for years, you can become more sensitive to pain. While people who take Kratom believe in its usefulness, many in the medical community judge that any benefits are offset by side effects and safety issues. Some sources, such as the Mayo Clinic, consider Kratom to be ineffective. However, the National Institutes of Health (NIH) reports that Kratom is increasingly recognized as a remedy for opioid withdrawal by individuals who self-treat for chronic pain.

Kratom has been reported to cause abnormal brain function when taken with prescription medicines. If you're taking any medication that warns you against drinking grapefruit juice, then you should avoid Kratom as well. The Food and Drug Administration (FDA) has warned about the dangers of Kratom and as of 2021 it is actually illegal in six states.

Tip #36: Voltaren

This used to be a prescription pain-relief product that is now available over the counter. It contains a very potent anti-inflammatory drug, diclofenac, which is a nonsteroidal or NSAID that can be absorbed through your skin. It works by reducing issues in the body that cause pain and inflammation, especially when they're caused by osteoarthritis, in the hands, wrists, knees, ankles and feet.

The product is available in a variety of forms including patch, solution, gel, spray and cream. It may take several days for you to feel significant pain relief. Do not use this product in larger amounts or for longer periods than recommended and try to use the lowest dose that's effective for you.

Do not use Voltaren if you've ever had an allergic reaction to aspirin, diclofenac or other NSAID or had asthma. Diclofenac can increase the risk of a fatal heart attack or stroke. It can also cause stomach and intestinal bleeding which can also be fatal and can occur without warning.

Do not apply it to any open or infected skin. Do not cover the treated area with a bandage or expose it to heat from a sauna, hot tub or heating pad. Don't even use cosmetics, sunscreens, lotions, insect repellant or any other medicated skin products in the same area. As I've said before, with this type of product avoid exposing the treated skin to heat, sunlight or even tanning beds.

Prescribed Solutions

Tip #37: Vicodin

This drug is actually a combination of two other drugs, acetaminophen and hydrocodone. While acetaminophen is an OTC drug commonly known as Tylenol, hydrocodone is an opioid medication. The combination increases the effectiveness of hydrocodone working in the brain to change how your body reacts to pain, so it's used for severe pain.

This medication can be effective and safe if used for a short period of time under a doctor's care. However, it has a high risk of being misused and can cause addiction, which means the patient needs more and more of it for the same result. Stopping it suddenly can ignite withdrawal. Methadone, Buprenorphine and Naltrexone can reduce withdrawal symptoms and help with the detoxification process. Naloxone is used to treat an opioid overdose.

Tip #38: Fentanyl

Often called the most dangerous drug in America, Fentanyl is a synthetic opioid medicine like morphine, heroin or oxycodone that's prescribed to treat moderate to severe pain. It is 100 times stronger than morphine and 50 times stronger than heroin. It's called a narcotic analgesic. Fentanyl has been around since 1960 but its use has exploded in the past decade with the increase in immigration on our Southern border, both illegal and legal, along with domestic manufacturing.

Fentanyl binds to the receptors in the brain that affect pain and emotions, which is why in addition to powerful pain relief it also causes euphoria. It comes in a variety of forms including patches, nasal sprays, sublingual tablets, injections and even lollipops. As with any opiate, there is a risk of dependency and addiction. That means you think you can't live without it and will do anything to get it. Just because there haven't been any drug addicts in your family doesn't mean you won't be the first. There's a reason Fentanyl kills more than 100,000 Americans every year so please be very, very careful if you take this drug.

Investigative journalist and author, Ben Westhoff, who chronicled the rise of the fentanyl epidemic in his book, *Fentanyl, Inc.*, said it wasn't until dealers realized they could make so much more money by cutting other drugs with fentanyl that it became sort of a supply-driven phenomenon.

Fortunately today we have Naloxone, also known as Narcan, and Kloxxado. Both come in nasal sprays and are safe medications to reverse an opioid overdose. There is also a Zimhi and Naloxone injection as possible overdose medications.

Tip #39: Physical Therapy

If you've ever had surgery or suffered from an injury, you're probably already familiar with this tip. Physical therapy, or PT, is about treating chronic and acute conditions and is a conservative approach to treatment. The good news is that anyone can benefit from PT and it can treat a wide variety of health problems. In fact, the Centers for Disease Control and Prevention recently suggested that PT was an effective option for managing pain instead of opioid medications.

Physical Therapy techniques can range from simple stretching to therapeutic exercises, hot and cold therapy, and massage. The goal is to ease pain and improve how you function to improve your life. These licensed professionals are called PTs or physiotherapists and since 2016 you had to graduate from an accredited higher education institution with a Doctor of Physical Therapy (DPT) degree in order to sit for the national exam. If you have a serious illness or injury a PT won't take the place of your doctors but they will work with them to guide your treatments. PTs often have assistants who are also trained and licensed to do different types of treatments.

Before you begin working with a PT you need to ask questions, lots of questions. Start with your PT's training and license, and about their success rate for your type of health problem. Be sure to check with your own insurance coverage to be sure physical therapy is covered. While some states don't require a referral from a physician to begin seeing a PT, many do.

When you start going to a PT, speak up if you feel pain or discomfort performing any exercise. Some pain is to be expected in order to regain muscle function, but don't believe them if they say what you're feeling is just normal or to be expected! I can tell you from personal experience that being knocked down to an assistant is a bad sign and if it hurts too much it isn't helping, it's just adding hurt to your existing problem. If they're professional they'll listen to you and adjust your exercise routine or even change the techniques being used for your treatment.

The good news is that physical therapy can do wonders to reduce your pain. One study examined people with chronic low back pain who had just started and found that early PT decreased opioid use both short and long term. Another research study on chronic low back pain found that opioids were prescribed less when patients were referred to physical therapy.

Tip #40: Stem Cell Injection

One of the more controversial therapies in this book is Stem Cell Injection or what's called Regenerative Medicine. Stem cells are the body's raw materials because they can divide into other cells. Stem Cell Therapy can be used to promote your body's natural ability to heal itself from cell function lost to aging, disease or injury. I'm sure you've heard of stem cell treatments for knees, back pain, arthritis, diabetes and even hair loss. The fact is, the only treatments approved by the Food & Drug Administration (FDA) are bone marrow transplants although there are lots of clinical trials available looking at Parkinson's and Alzheimer's disease and Multiple Sclerosis (MS).

There are different types of stem cells, beginning with embryonic stem cells, from embryos that are three to five days old. Perinatal stem cells can be found in amniotic fluid and in umbilical cord blood. Adult stem cells exist in small numbers in most adult tissues but they have a more limited ability to grow into various cells in the body.

Some clinics sell stem cell therapy without FDA approval and this places the patient at a higher risk for side effects and poor outcomes. Please ask your health care provider to confirm if your treatment is approved. You can also ask the clinical investigator to give you the FDA-issued Investigational New Drug Application number and the chance to review the FDA communication acknowledging the IND. Ask for this information *before* getting treatment—even if the stem cells are your own. Be aware that unproven stem cell treatments can cost tens of thousands of dollars and aren't covered by insurance.

Tip #41: Placebo

After a dubious listing on Stem Cells, I thought it appropriate to follow up with the listing on the Placebo Effect. This comes from the Latin phrase "I shall please" and is used to describe the body's ability to heal itself. This completely natural type of healing should be the goal of every person, since this type of healing has no side effects and no toxic chemicals. One of the first research reports on the process was *The Powerful Placebo* (1955), and it concluded that an average of 32% of patients responded to the placebo.

Research today with the newest technology is unlocking many of the secrets of the placebo effect but it's also creating even more questions about this powerful human ability. Researchers in Italy have discovered that there isn't one placebo effect but many different types. Researchers in the U.S. have found that the process isn't simply a psychological phenomenon as originally thought but is a real, physical response to belief and expectation. Neuroscientist, Helen Mayberg, discovered in 2002 that inert pills (placebos) work the same way on the brains of depressed people as antidepressants.

Activity in the seat of higher thought, the frontal cortex, increased while activity in the area for emotions, the limbic regions, decreased.

Anatomy of Hope (2003) by Harvard Medical School physician, Jerome Groopman, M.D. says that "A change of mindset can alter neurochemistry both in a laboratory setting and in the clinic." Dr. Groopman experienced the power of the placebo effect releasing the brain's endorphins and enkephlins to relieve his own back pain, which is why it's included in a book on chronic pain.

The Allen Brain Atlas, founded by Microsoft co-founder Paul Allen, was completed in 2006. The project researched where each gene was activated in a mouse's brain because of its many similarities to human brains. They discovered that 80% of the 21,000 genes in a mouse body were activated in the brain, more than anyone expected. This is a possible indication of the scope of the mind-body connection and the power of the placebo effect. This may also be a window into the function of epigenetics.

Medically inactive pills, often called sugar pills, are used to simulate real medications during testing of new medications to determine if they're more effective than the placebo effect. A new product that can't produce positive results higher than the placebo will not be approved by the Food and Drug Administration (FDA). The pharmaceutical industry has successfully tainted the term "placebo effect" with a very negative connotation, because to them it's a real problem with financial consequences. However it should be remembered that it is a powerful healing process. Because it can't be patented and sold for a profit, this all-natural healing capacity has a negative effect on the modern drug industry but a very positive effect on patients.

Unfortunately for the drug industry, the rate of positive responses to placebos have improved over the years as a result of better test design and the use of so-called active placebos that provide a detectable response unrelated to the problem. The better the placebo response, the more difficult it is for new drugs to demonstrate effectiveness.

The good news for anyone suffering with chronic pain is that you may have your own pain solution within you right now. The challenge is how to tap into this hidden asset for your own relief.

Tip #42: Injections

Millions of Americans suffer from joint pain and many have made the trip to the doctor's office for an injection. There are several different types of injections, starting with corticosteroids, or steroids for short. Steroid shots can be very effective, especially for the later stages of arthritis, at least for a few weeks. If cortisone shots don't work, your doctor may try a Hyaluronic acid (HA) or gel injection for knee pain.

One of the newer injection options is platelet-rich plasma (PRP). Cells from your own blood are processed to remove red and white blood cells to concentrate the plasma, which your doctor will inject the following day.

An even newer option is Autologous conditioned serum (ACS), which is also made from your own blood in a manner similar to platelet-rich plasma. This option is only done by specialists and can range from a single-shot treatment to several shots over a few weeks. This isn't usually covered by insurance, so you may be paying thousands of dollars for this type of pain relief.

There are also stem cell injections using material collected either from your bone marrow or fat cells. Unfortunately, the number of actual stem cells injected in incredibly small and results have not lived up to the hype.

Common side effects for injection shots range from pain at the injection site to bruising, swelling, redness on the skin and even a temporary increase in blood sugar levels.

Tip #43: Tramadol

Wow. The list of the possible very serious side effects and damage to your body are very, very long with this drug. To say that it has serious warnings from the FDA is a huge understatement. Tramadol is a controlled substance, which means it must only be used under the very close supervision of your doctor. This is an opioid agonist medicine that changes how your brain perceives pain. It's similar to the substances in your brain called endorphins that bind to the nerve receptors to decrease the pain messages your body sends your brain. While effective to treat moderate and severe pain, it can easily become habit forming, especially with prolonged usage.

Tramadol can cause serious breathing problems, especially during the first 24 - 72 hours when you begin taking it, or any time your dose is increased. It comes as an oral tablet in both a generic and the brand name of Ultram in immediate and extended-release forms.

Be aware that Tramadol can lead to opioid addiction or abuse. This drug can dramatically slow or even stop your breathing. If you take it with benzodiazepines or other CNS depressants like alcohol, it can cause serious side effects, many of which can be life-threatening.

As I said, the list of warnings is very long, including to not take if you have asthma or other breathing problems, any stomach or bowel obstruction, if you've recently used alcohol, sedatives or tranquilizers or even if you've used an MAO inhibitor in the past 14 days. Please check with your doctor about all of the medications and OTC supplements you're currently using before beginning treatment with Tramadol.

Tip #44: Medical Marijuana or Cannabis

While this may help your chronic pain it can also get you in trouble with the law. While the federal government prohibits the use of marijuana, more than two thirds of our states and the District of Columbia have legalized it for medical treatments. Be aware that federal law regulating marijuana supersedes state laws, which means folks have been arrested and charged with possession even in states where marijuana is legal.

Medical marijuana or cannabis is the term used for derivatives of the Cannabis sativa plant. There are over 100 different chemicals or cannabinoids in it, but the best known are the delta-9 tetrahydro-cannabinol (THC), which is what gets people "high" and cannabidiol (CBD), which usually comes from the hemp plant for medical use.

Qualifying for medical marijuana will depend on what state you live in. You will have to meet certain requirements if you have a qualifying condition such as Alzheimer's disease, glaucoma, severe or chronic pain and other conditions. The good news is that some of the best research on the therapeutic effects of cannabis relates to its ability to reduce chronic pain and relieve inflammation.

Medical marijuana is available in a variety of forms including: capsules, liquid, oil, powder and, dried leaves. This means you have many options on how to use it such as:

- Smoking it
- Using a vaporizer to inhale it
- Eat in in a brownie or lollipop
- Apply it to your skin in a lotion or cream
- Place a few drops of the liquid under your tongue.

Be warned that you should use medical cannabis with extra caution, especially if you have a history of substance misuse, psychosis or cardiac arrhythmias.

Tip #45: Oxycodone

As long as I'm warning you about the use of some of these therapies, I'll add a huge word of caution about the use of the prescription drug Oxycontin and Oxycodone. You may have heard about Oxycontin from the Purdue Pharma settlement announced on September 1, 2021, where the Sackler family agreed to pay $4.3 billion to mitigate Oxycontin misuse along with forfeiting ownership of the company. The family had made more than $10 billion selling Oxycontin. The settlement came after the worst year (2020) of opioid overdose deaths with over 93,000 dying.

Oxycodone is an immediate-release, generic drug sold under many names including Xtampza ER, Oxaydo and Roxybond. Oxycontin is the brand name of the extended-release version of the drug. This is a morphine-like drug for strong pain relief. Both versions bind to receptors in your brain and spinal cord to block pain signals. It comes in a tablet, capsule or liquid form.

If you're going to take this medication, do so only on a regular schedule as prescribed by your doctor. This is not meant to be used for breakthrough or sudden pain. Do not drink alcohol while taking it because the combination can be fatal. Avoid eating grapefruit or drinking grapefruit juice while on this medication because it can increase the chance of side effects.

Most important, be aware that this medication can cause addiction (long-term physical or psychological dependence). Suddenly stopping it can cause withdrawal so work with your doctor to reduce your dose slowly.

Tip #46: Percocet

This is another one of those combination drugs, this time it's oxycodone and acetaminophen. It's still a dangerous narcotic that can cause addiction. It comes in a tablet, capsule, extended-release tablet and capsule and even a liquid for those who have trouble swallowing pills. If you take extended-release pills or tablets, be sure to swallow them whole, don't break, divide, crush, presoak or dissolve them in any way. If you take the liquid form, use a medication-measuring device and not a spoon to be sure you're getting the prescribed amount.

Be aware that during the first 24-72 hours of your treatment or when your dose is increased, it can cause life-threatening breathing problems. You shouldn't use Percocet if you've recently used alcohol, sedatives, tranquilizers or other opioid medications. If you've used an MAO inhibiter in the past two weeks don't use Percocet. Percocet interacts with many other products like cold and allergy medicines, bronchodilator or COPD medications, even a diuretic. Sedatives like Valium are also a problem. Even St. John's wort and tryptophan can cause problems. Be sure and avoid eating grapefruit or drinking grapefruit juice while taking this medication unless your doctor says it's safe to do so.

This medication can cause addiction. Never take Percocet in larger amounts or for longer than your doctor prescribes. Finally, you should know that Percocet may decrease fertility in both men and women.

Tip #47: Ubrelvy

As long as we're talking about headaches, Ubrelvy is a calcitonin gene-related peptide antagonist (CGRP inhibitor) to treat migraine headaches in adults, but it will not prevent them. It was approved by the FDA in 2019. As always with a prescription drug, you need to tell your doctor about all of your other prescriptions, non-prescription drugs and even the herbal products you take. It's available in either 50mg or 100mg size tablets. It is not a narcotic and does not cause addiction. Also be sure to tell your doctor if you have liver or kidney disease before you start taking this medication.

You shouldn't take it if you're already taking CYP3A4 Inhibitors like Ketoconazole, Clarithromysin or Itraconazole. You should also avoid it if you're taking Nefazodone, clarithromycin, telithromycin, itraconazole or antiviral medications to treat HIV/AIDS.

If your headache doesn't go away after your first dose of Ubrelvy, you can take a second tablet if it's been at least two hours since your first dose.

Thinking About It

Tip #48: Humor Therapy

It's often been said by those outside the mainstream medical community that "laughter may indeed be the best medicine," possibly because it's affordable but also because it's true. Humor Therapy is often considered a type of Psychoneuroimmunology.

Doctors didn't seriously consider laughter a legitimate form of therapy until the New England Journal of Medicine published the Norman Cousins case study in 1979 showing how laughter could reverse a serious disease. Norman Cousins published *Anatomy of an Illness* in 1964 about his fight with ankylosing spondylitis, a painful disintegration of the connective tissue in the spine. He designed his own humor therapy and discovered that 15 minutes of laughter could bring him up to two hours of pain-free sleep. Since that time laughter has been found to lower blood pressure, reduce stress hormones, boost immune system function and release endorphins, the body's natural painkillers. A good belly laugh is considered a type of exercise providing good cardiac conditioning for those unable to perform regular physical exercise. Best of all, it produces a wonderful sense of wellbeing. It's also a great coping mechanism and is increasingly used for the treatment of cancer.

Today, doctors are often still afraid to use humor. There is no reference to humor therapy in most medical training manuals or programs. There has been very little research because humor can't be patented and no research means there are no articles in professional journals. Doctors may also be concerned that it may reduce the professional distance from the patient. All of these are "old school" problems that are slowly fading away as the overwhelming benefits of humor become more accepted.

One example is the Big Apple Circus in New York, which created Clown Care twenty years ago to entertain children. Today they have 84 professional clowns working at hospitals in cities across the country. New York Presbyterian Hospital has these clowns working at the Morgan Stanley Children's Hospital three days each week all year long. Many other hospitals are implementing Comedy Crash Carts for laughter emergencies and adding the Chuckle Channel to their TV channel selection to improve the quality of life of their patients.

Many years ago, Dr. Madan Kataria in India created Laughter Yoga as a result of his research on laughter. Today there are thousands of Laughter Clubs and other groups around the world to spread the benefits of laughter. One of the most important benefits is that you live in the moment. Focusing on the beauty of life right now has many wonderful effects.

The Association for Applied and Therapeutic Humor (AATH) was created in 1987 to "advance the understanding and application of humor and laughter for their positive benefits." It is an international community of professionals who incorporate humor into their daily lives.

Tip #49: Hypnosis

Clinical Hypnosis is a state of mind where communication with the subconscious is enabled while bypassing the conscious mind. It has also been called a state of focused concentration. While there is general agreement about some of the effects of hypnosis, there are a variety of definitions of hypnosis and many different theories about how and why it works. If you've ever driven several miles and not known how you got there, you've experienced a type of hypnosis called highway hypnosis. It's a similar sensation to reading a book intently or focusing completely on a TV program so that you become unaware of your surroundings.

There are three major styles of hypnosis: Suggestion, Mental Imagery, and Self. The first type is where a trained hypnotist speaks softly and rhythmically to produce an enhanced state of relaxation.

With the second style the hypnotist talks about specific scenes to produce focused concentration. The third type is self-induced.

Hypnotherapy or clinical hypnosis is often used to treat conditions such as phobias, anxiety, and chronic pain. It's also used for age regression therapy, enhancing self-esteem and improving memory and concentration. It's been used in medicine for anesthesia and for childbirth along with other conditions. Hypnosis is even used by dentists to control fear, saliva and gagging. Lay hypnotists use it to help clients stop smoking, to lose weight, and to activate the mind-body connection to aid in the treatment of fibromyalgia, cancer, diabetes and arthritis.

Franz Anton Mesmer, a charismatic healer, developed the forerunner of modern hypnosis in the 18th century but the basic principles have been around for thousands of years. James Braid coined the term hypnosis in 1843 referring to Hypnos, the Greek god of sleep because of the resemblance of mesmerism to sleep. Modern hypnosis is due to pioneers like Clark Hull and his student, Milton Erickson. Ericksonian Hypnosis uses a passive technique to work with the subconscious instead of the regular commanding style. The American Medical Association approved the use of hypnosis in 1958 and the American Psychological Association accepted it in 1960.

Many people confuse stage hypnotism with hypnotherapy, failing to appreciate that stage hypnotists screen their volunteers to select the most cooperative candidates, possibly with exhibitionist tendencies. This type of entertainment perpetuates a myth about hypnosis which discourages people from seeking legitimate hypnotherapy.

Tip #50: Prayer Therapy

According to the 2002 study by the federal government, 45% of Americans have used prayer for health reasons. However, the 2007 survey chose not to include prayer therapy. Prayer Therapy is a process of learning how to pray effectively by combining the insights of psychology with the power of prayer. Prayer is considered vital to our lives because each person needs to communicate with his or her God in order to reach their full potential.

Prayer Therapy began with a grant in the 1950s to William R. Parker, Ph.D. from the Religion in Education Foundation to compare the effectiveness of prayer, psychotherapy and a combination of the two processes. *Prayer Can Change Your Life* by Dr. Parker and Elaine St. Johns reports on this research.

Prayer can be words, thoughts or images but they express inspiration, devotion and affirmation. As an alternative to psycho-therapy, Prayer Therapy is a systematic process of discovering hidden insights and the power of the soul for personal growth. It is based on the belief that every human being has a body, mind and soul and that while changing thinking or behavior can be beneficial, prayer can be a healing tonic for the soul.

Prayer Therapy must be practiced with honesty and love to be effective, which can be very challenging. Honesty is difficult because we all want to support our own perspective because we see it as being in our own best interest. Love is the healing power but it can also be a challenge for many people.

Different methods may be used to progress through stages of development. Prayer Therapy practitioners may be ministers, medical professionals, or simply lay people. Today Amplified Prayer Therapy (APT) connects the world of prayer with quantum science.

The works of Dr. Masaru Emoto, a Japanese scientist, are often used to support this new approach. His movie "What The Bleep Do We Know," and his book *The True Power of Water* offer evidence that physical items like molecules of water may be affected by the energy of our thoughts, words, feelings, and even our music. This means that our prayers literally have the power not only to change who we are but also to change the world around us.

Tip #51: EFT or Emotional Freedom Technique

EFT was developed in the early 1990s by Stanford engineer Gary Craig based on the Thought Field Transfer (*TFT*) process. Basically, it's an American innovation on the concepts of acupressure. The fundamental principle is that negative emotions produce an upset in the body's energy system, which can be corrected by applying pressure or "tapping" on the major energy meridians. The Basic EFT process employs a comprehensive sequence of tapping points to cover all problems. Tapping, as it's also called, uses the fingertips to tap on fourteen different points on the body to stimulate all of the major energy meridians. The Basic Recipe is called a ham sandwich of steps: Set-Up; the Basic Sequence (13 steps); the 9 Gamut step, and then another round of Basic Sequence. The entire process usually takes less than two minutes and can be learned very quickly. Follow-up rounds of EFT may be abbreviated with various shortcut routines using modified Set-Up and Reminder phrases. This process is designed for people to use by themselves but there are many experienced facilitators available for more challenging problems, either in person or by telephone.

The success of EFT has also created a growing range of variations and derivatives such as the Active Choice Technique, Creating and Receiving Technique, the Healing and Release Technique, the Light Imagery Grateful Heart Technique, the Miracle Acupressure Tapping Technique and many, many others.

Tip #52: PSYCH-K®

If the drugs you're taking aren't working well enough or if your doctor scratches his head because he doesn't understand your chronic pain, it may be time to look at it differently. We know that the brain is where we actually feel pain, so we have to consider that our brain, in particular our subconscious, may be its source. Working with your subconscious to resolve your pain is a very different problem.

Originally called Psychological Kinesiology, PSYCH-K® uses muscle testing or Applied Kinesiology to work directly with the subconscious mind. Many health issues and problems can be traced to subconscious beliefs. Developed in the late 1980s, it is based on the formula:

Beliefs=Thoughts/Feelings=Actions=Reality.

The PSYCH-K® process is a unique method to locate problem subconscious beliefs and quickly transform them into beliefs that support your best life, which means no more chronic pain. These subconscious beliefs function like filters distorting our view of life and ourselves. By changing subconscious beliefs to support our best life, we can dramatically improve our lives. Beliefs that have been held for years or decades can be changed in minutes with this technique.

The process uses the straight-arm style of muscle testing with light to moderate pressure by the facilitator. The goal is to obtain either a "lock" or "unlock" response to a statement spoken by either the facilitator or client. A locked or straight arm indicates a yes/positive response while a weak or unlocked arm is a no/negative answer.

Tip #53: Mindfulness Based Stress Reduction

Mindfulness Based Stress Reduction is more than the name implies. It is a process of intentionally focused awareness of the present moment without judgment as a method of self-reflection. MBSR operates without the restrictive attitudes of yourself, others or the world. When Jon Kabat-Zinn, Ph.D. began a new type of alternative health program at the University of Massachusetts Medical School in 1979 he called it the Stress Reduction Clinic because meditation was considered too "far out" to be taken seriously at the time. As news of his results spread throughout the hospital, more difficult cases were referred to him and his success continued to grow. The program became more accepted and continued to expand, eventually becoming The Center for Mindfulness in Medicine, Healthcare and Society.

Today the program is a course of eight weekly classes with one full day of class on a Saturday or Sunday. It includes gentle stretching and mindful Yoga exercises along with guided instruction into methods of mindfulness meditation. There are also exercises to improve awareness of everyday life, group dialogue, individual instruction and daily homework assignments using tapes and workbooks. It's a challenging but life-affirming process as participants learn to relate to what's happening in their lives in a positive new way by learning how to take charge. The process also teaches you how to do what no one else can do for you—consciously and systematically work through your own stress, pain, illness or other life challenges.

MBSR also taps directly into the spiritual discipline of the heart, spirit, soul, Tao, Dharma or other entity name. This type of present-moment awareness helps you to experience your life not only with acceptance but also an eager curiosity and appreciation. Participants learn to open their eyes to the pleasures of their life and improve their skills for tapping into their own wisdom and internal resources.

There have been decades of research on MBSR since the program's inception documenting the many benefits of the process. Participants increase their ability to relax, and experience decreases in physical problems like pain and psychological symptoms with a corresponding increase in self-esteem, energy and enthusiasm for life.

Today, more than 13,000 people have completed the MBSR program and there are more than 300 trained practitioners involved in programs at hundreds of hospitals around the country. The program has been featured in the Bill Moyers' PBS documentary *Healing and the Mind,* on Oprah, NBC's *Dateline*, ABC's *Chronicle* and in other programs and articles. Jon Kabat-Zinn's book *Full Catastrophe Living* provides an introduction to mindfulness training. For people who cannot afford it, or cannot physically attend, David Potter runs a free online version that is certified by Jon Kabatt-Zinn, see https://palousemindfulness.com.

Tip #54: Mindfulness

Mindfulness is becoming intentionally aware of your thoughts and actions in the present moment in a totally non-judgmental manner. It has been around for thousands of years and is a fundamental part of Buddhism but today Western therapists are also embracing it as an effective way to deal with depression, anxiety and even pain.

Mindfulness is simply being aware of your present moment without judging or thinking, you simply are "in the moment" completely. It's been said that a moment is like a breath because both are replaced by the next one. An ancient Japanese saying explains it as: "Wherever you go, there you are." Mindfulness is a way to accept that the past is history and nothing can change it, while the future is not here yet, so there is no need to fear it. Being "in the moment" helps us to appreciate that the gift of life is right now as a way to help us control our pain.

Mindfulness does not have to be limited to a formal meditation session, but can be done at any time in almost any way because it is simply bringing the mind into focus on the present moment. If you're walking and notice the feel of the ground underneath your feet, the wind on your face and everything going on around you, you're practicing a type of mindfulness.

A more formal style of Mindfulness in meditation is to give a label to each breath in and out to help concentrate attention on the moment and to disregard the mind's usual running commentary. Mindfulness can bring about an awareness that happiness isn't brought about by a change in your external situation, it originates inside.

There are two different types of mindful meditation in Buddhism called Vipassana and Samatha. Vipassana is translated as "insight" or the full awareness of what is happening as it happens. Samatha is considered "concentration" or tranquility, that state when the mind is brought to rest and not allowed to wander. When it does wander, you acknowledge the intrusion, even thank it, then gently return your attention to your chosen focus. Most systems of meditation focus on Samatha and use a prayer, candle or other device to exclude all other thoughts.

It's interesting to note that one of the first applications of Mindfulness in England was to help with pain. A patient by the name of Vidyamala Burch found it helped with her own severe, chronic pain. After experiencing success in 2000, she started

Breathworks to help others with their chronic pain with an eight-week course that has now been taught to thousands of participants in over twenty countries.

Tip #55: Meditation

Since all of your pain registers in your brain, we have to explore all of the possible mental therapies and treatments. The term "Meditation" has different meanings to different people. It's used to describe a wide range of practices with many different goals but we generally associate the term with focusing our attention inward. It is used most often to relieve stress and provide a feeling of peace. It can also be used for personal or spiritual development and for healing and relief from chronic pain.

Meditation comes from a variety of Eastern traditions and there are a variety of techniques involved in meditation depending on the spiritual tradition and/or practitioner (see also Prayer Therapy). Meditation can involve focusing on a specific object, on the background, or shifting between the two. Postures may be sitting, lying down, kneeling or sitting cross-legged. In almost every case the spine should be kept straight for proper energy flow. Time requirements also vary widely but generally 20-30 minutes per day is accepted as a normal amount of time for meditation.

Transcendental Meditation® (also called TM) is one of its most recognized forms . This is the program of Maharishi Mahesh Yogi, which promotes two twenty-minute sessions of meditation each day in a seated position with eyes closed. Training involves the awarding of a unique mantra for each individual to fully experience the restful alertness of the process. The technique is taught in a four-day course with a 90-minute session each day. Most of the research on the health effects of meditation has been done on TM.

Another style of meditation is called the Relaxation Response after the 1975 book by Herbert Benson, M.D., Associate Professor of Medicine at the Harvard Medical School. Separating the beneficial effects of meditation from religious connotations, Dr. Benson's research showed that repetition of a sound, word, phrase or even movement and simply putting intruding thoughts aside could create what he termed the Relaxation Response. This was the counterbalance to our stress response, also called the fight-or-flight response, which is a frequent result of pain.

Tip #56: EMDR (Eye Movement Desensitization and Reprocessing)

EMDR barely qualifies as "alternative therapy" today due to its proven effectiveness and wide acceptance by established medicine, but it is still new enough to be considered outside the mainstream by some. Francine Shapiro discovered in 1987 that eye movements appeared to decrease the negative emotions connected with distressing memories. Increased stress and tension can cause all sorts of pain and discomfort. Eye movements alone did not create a comprehensive therapeutic effect, so she added other treatment elements and developed a standard procedure called Eye Movement Desensitization, changing the name in 1991 as a result of further development.

EMDR is an information-processing therapy that integrates elements of several different psychotherapies for maximum effect. These include psychodynamic, cognitive-behavioral, interpersonal, experiential, and body-centered therapies which are used in an eight-phase sequence. The process uses standardized procedures that include having the client remember difficult or traumatic experiences while simultaneously focusing on an external stimulus such as following the therapist's fingers back and forth with their eyes for 20 or 30 seconds. Therapists also use sounds, tapping or other touch stimulation in this therapy.

Research studies have shown the process very effective in treating traumatic disorders, even Post Traumatic Stress Disorder (PTSD). In 2004, the American Psychiatric Association gave their highest level of recommendation to EMDR for the treatment of trauma. That same year the Department of Veterans Affairs classified EMDR as "strongly recommended."

Training is intended only for licensed or qualified mental health professionals such as graduate students under the supervision of a licensed professional. In the U.S., the EMDR Institute, where Francine Shapiro, Ph.D. is the Executive Director, offers training. Certification is done by the EMDR International Association (EMDRIA).

Tip #57: Cognitive-Behavioral Therapy (CBT)

Cognitive-Behavioral Therapy (CBT) is a type of psychotherapy built on the principle that changing the way a person thinks will also change their behavior and how they feel. The client is an active participant in this correction process for faulty learning experiences and distorted thinking. By recognizing and then correcting negative thoughts and dysfunctional attitudes a new, more positive and productive perspective can reshape their life.

The process begins with a full medical/treatment history of the problem. Next a detailed record is made by the patient of each episode so that common factors can be identified. Once a clear picture of the problem or condition is obtained, the patient is then given techniques to better ground themselves so they can be more in control of their situation. These normally include various types of relaxation techniques. The next step in the process is Cognitive Restructuring or learning what thoughts trigger the problem so new, more positive thoughts can take their place.

CBT has a collection of about fifty different methods to choose from today. All-or-nothing thinking is one example of erroneous thinking processes with its own healing method. Looking through the wrong end of the telescope is another thinking error. In this situation the patient focuses on one problem or small part of their life, neglecting the rest of reality. This type of obsessive condition makes perfect sense to the patient because it's all they can see, but others cannot understand how they can ignore everything. With recognition of the thinking error and the proper correction technique, healing can be rapid and long-lasting.

While normally considered a type of therapy used by trained psychotherapists, there are also self-help CBT options available. *Feeling Good: The New Mood Therapy* by David D. Burns and Aaron T. Beck was first published in 1980 and it's a wonderful primer on identifying and correcting the distorted thinking involved in depression and other disorders. They were among the first to say the history of a problem wasn't as important to the patient as changing it in the here and now. This attitude began a revolution in traditional talk therapy. It is often considered an alternative type of therapy even today. Research studies are underway involving CBT for several conditions. CBT has an 85% success rate, about the same as surgery for various physical conditions. MRI studies have shown that it produces the same brain changes as antidepressants with the added benefit of being drug-free.

The Beck Depression Inventory (BDI, BDI-II) is a twenty-one-question test created by Dr. Aaron T. Beck to measure the severity of depression. The first version was published in 1961, revised in 1971 and the BDI-II was published in 1996. It is considered a standard evaluation tool for many conditions.

Since all pain comes from nerves, how we think will also change how we feel, critically important for those who suffer from chronic pain. To put this into perspective, it helps to remember the story of two different pain sufferers and how they react to their pain. The first person suffers pain 24/7 and hasn't found anything to help relieve the symptoms so their life is sad and terrible. The second person suffers pain 24/7 but lives a full and active life because they're able to deal with their pain on their own. How? They simply tell their pain to go sit in a chair in the corner. By taking control of their pain and telling it where it should be they're free to live their life. Chronic pain is all about nerves and nerves can be controlled.

Medical Solutions

Tip #58: Acupuncture

Acupuncture is estimated to be around 5,000 years old and is a vital part of Traditional Chinese Medicine (TCM). The technique stems from the belief that the body's vital energy Chi or Qi (pronounced chee) flows throughout the human body and all of nature.

Chi travels throughout the body along meridians or channels. The meridians mirror themselves in pairs on both sides of the body. There are fourteen primary meridians running vertically up and down the surface of the body. Each half of the body has twelve main or organ meridians along with eight secondary and two unpaired midline meridians.

There are more than 2,000 acupuncture points or specific locations where the meridians come to the surface of the skin, so practitioners can easily reach them with one of the nine types of acupuncture needles (but they commonly only use six in America today and the good news is they're thinner than those used in China). The connections between acupuncture points ensure that there is an even circulation of Chi creating a balance between yin and yang. Energy constantly flows up and down these pathways, but there is a problem whenever the pathways become too strong, too weak, obstructed or just unbalanced. Acupuncture restores the balance. There are also different devices and types of acupuncture. A Plum Blossom is the "hitting hammer," because the device has a group of needles on its surface for a different acupuncture effect.

Acupressure is simply acupuncture without needles. The practitioner uses a hand, knuckle or a small device to stimulate the acupuncture points. There is also Moxibustion, which is applying heat to acupuncture points. Cupping is a technique that uses suction, frequently created by warming a glass cup, to draw blood to a site for stimulation.

There are also complementary types of treatments to acupuncture. Auricular acupuncture involves only the points in the ear. Newer variations include using cold lasers to stimulate acupuncture points using different types of lasers to reach different depths. Acupuncture can also be done using sound waves (sonupuncture) to stimulate acupuncture points. Using colored lights to stimulate acupuncture points is called colorpuncture.

In 2005, a combined study by the National Institute of Health and The Mayo Clinic confirmed that acupuncture can help relieve the pain of fibromyalgia and can be a beneficial complement to treatments for osteoarthritis of the knee. Clearly your pain may benefit from acupuncture.

Tip #59: Osteopathic Medicine

Osteopathic Medicine or Osteopathy is a holistic approach to healthcare recognizing the unity of all body parts and the body's ability to heal itself. A U.S. Army doctor, Andrew Taylor Still, M.D., founded Osteopathy in 1874. In this philosophy of health, a human being is more than simply the sum of its body parts. Osteopathy is considered a separate but equal branch of medical care in this country, having become integrated with mainstream medicine in 1969. However, outside the U.S., where it has remained essentially a drug free system based on manipulative techniques, it is still considered a complementary process in the USA.

Doctors of Osteopathy, or D.O.s, receive full medical training of four years of medical school, three to six years of internship or residency and additional training just like mainstream or allopathic physicians. D.O.s receive extra training in the musculoskeletal system, the relationship between the muscles, bones and nerves, so they better understand how a problem in one part of the body can impact other areas.

D.O.s are trained to use their hands to help diagnose and treat injury and illness using osteopathic manipulative treatment or OMT.

This involves moving the muscles and joints with stretching, resistance and the gentle use of pressure to properly align the body. However they also recognize that sometimes medication and surgery may be required therapy.

These are the eight generally accepted principles of osteopathy including concepts like "the body is a unit" and "structure and function are interrelated." They appreciate how body fluids are essential to health and that nerves play a vital role in the motion of fluids. The body can heal itself but maintaining health today is a constant struggle against stress, environmental toxins and other challenges. They believe in a holistic approach to health to prevent illness.

After enduring the horrors of the Civil War battlefield and then the loss of his wife and children from disease, Dr. Still lost his faith in the standard medicine of the day. Conventional medicine at that time was using mercury as medicine. He began researching and testing other methods of healing and in 1892 founded the American School of Osteopathy in Kirksville, Missouri, as the first medical school of its kind in the world. His methods attracted a great deal of unpleasant attention at the time and Kirksville was one of the few places that allowed him to practice. Today it's called Andrew Taylor Still University, Kirksville College of Osteopathic Medicine. Although Missouri was willing to grant him a charter for awarding medical doctor degrees, he was so unhappy with the field that he chose to issue his own D.O. degree.

Both Doctors of Osteopathy and Medical Doctors must pass comparable examinations to obtain state licenses to practice medicine and work in fully accredited and licensed healthcare facilities.

Tip #60: Homeopathy

You may not have heard of Homeopathy or Homeotherapeutics, but it is a complete system of medicine based on the Law of Similars, or "let likes be cured by likes." It takes a holistic perspective of people and illness with the goal of promoting optimal health. According to the World Health Organization, it is the second most practiced form of medicine in the world today.

In this system, an illness is simply the body's attempt to heal itself and homeopathic remedies trigger the body's self-healing abilities by increasing the life force and correcting imbalances. The process stimulates an accelerated immune system response and releases underlying energetic blocks by using minute amounts of substances that serve as a catalyst to the body. These substances may be from plants, minerals, animals or even from chemical drugs, but are carefully diluted until very little of the original is left in the solution. All homeopathic medicines are made with the processes described in the official manufacturing manual called the *Homeopathic Pharmacopoeia of the United States*, which is recognized by the FDA.

Homeopathy was first theorized by Hippocrates, but it was German doctor, C. F. Samuel Hahnemann, who is credited with its first practical application in 1796. It was brought to the U.S. around 1825 by doctors trained in Europe and by 1900 there were an estimated 22 homeopathic medical colleges. Estimates were that 20% of U.S. doctors used homeopathy at that time. However, the move toward the mechanical model of the human body pushed homeopathy out of the mainstream.

Homeopathy has been proven to be more effective than main-stream (allopathic) medicine in the treatment and prevention of disease without harmful side effects. In a frequently quoted bit of American history, it's reported that the cholera outbreak in 1849 saw allopathic medicine produce death rates of 48-60% while homeopathic hospitals had a death rate of only 3%.

Homeopathy is much more accepted and popular in the rest of the world. For example, there are more than 300 homeopathic medical colleges in India. In the U.K., 42% of physicians refer patients to homeopaths and in France 25% of physicians use homeopathy in their practice.

There was new research in 2009, showing that homeopathic solutions may be effective even though they've been diluted many times. The winner of the Nobel Prize in 2008, Prof. Luc Montagnier, reported that a series of rigorous experiments demonstrated that electromagnetic properties remain in highly diluted biological samples. Dr. Montagnier is a French virologist, who co-discovered HIV. Homeopathy was not mentioned specifically in the paper but the process was similar because they used aqueous solutions that were agitated and serially diluted, noting that the strong agitation was critical for the generation of electromagnetic signals. Anyone familiar with homeopathy recognizes the traditional homeopathic distillation process.

Sequential Homeopathy is a relatively recent development in the field to address multiple blockages or problems. It uses multiple remedies to reverse the chronological layers causing each problem. Practitioners see clients every 1-2 months because each layer requires 4-8 weeks to release its toxins and heal the affected organs and systems. This process is often used to treat allergies, autism spectrum disorders and auto-immune diseases where the body is attacking itself to recover from toxicity contained in the cells.

The American Institute of Homeopathy was established in 1844 and remains the oldest national medical profession in the United States. Another organization representing all professional homeopaths in North America is the North American Society of Homeopaths (NASH). The National Center for Homeopathy has offered instruction in homeopathy for more than 70 years. There are many training programs in homeopathy, but no certificate is recognized as a license to practice homeopathy in the USA. Laws regarding homeopathy vary widely from state to state but normally it can be practiced legally by licensed medical professionals. New health freedom laws are increasingly permitting it to be practiced by non-licensed professionals as well, so check to see what regulations apply where you live. In addition, homeopathic remedies are sold over the counter for self-care.

Tip #61: Ayurveda

Ayurveda in Sanskrit means "The Science of Life" and it's believed to be more than 5,000 years old, making it one of the oldest health systems in the world. Developed in India, Ayurvedic medicine focuses on developing a balance of mind, body and spirit to maintain health and prevent illness. Each person is unique, with an individual energy signature, their own mix of physical, mental and emotional characteristics. Proper thinking, lifestyle, diet and herbs are used to achieve proper balance for each person. Creating and maintaining proper health in your body will reduce (and hopefully eliminate) your chronic pain. There are many similarities between Ayurveda and Traditional Chinese Medicine (TCM).

The vital energy of a person is called Prana, which is centered around the energy centers in the body called Chakras. Unlike the Traditional Chinese system of Yin/Yang, the Indian energy system has three separate elements or doshas:

- Vata Dosha, composed of space and air; it is the energy of movement.
- Patta Dosha is made of fire and water; it's the body's metabolic processes.
- Kapha Dosha is the glue that holds it together, the body's structure represented by earth and water.

Ayurveda uses a holistic approach with therapies that appeal to all of the senses to treat each individual. Practitioners may use Taste (herbs and nutrition); Touch (massage, yoga, exercise); Smell (aromatherapy); Sight (color therapy); Hearing (music therapy, mantra meditation, chanting) and Spiritual therapy. The system is about more than just health, it's about living.

Tip #62: Qi Gong or QiGong

Qi Gong (pronounced chee-kung) combines motion and meditation by simultaneously performing postures, breathing techniques, and focused intentions. "Qi" means breath or the energy produced by breathing, and "gong" means work or skill, so QiGong can mean "breath work" or "skill of attracting vital energy." The practice is said to go back up to 5,000 years in China and is considered part of Traditional Chinese Medicine, which is why it's beneficial for chronic pain relief. Chinese hospitals have officially recognized Medical QiGong treatment as a standard medical technique since 1989.

There are an estimated 3,000+ different styles and schools of Qigong but the various practices can be classified as a martial art, medical or spiritual practice. All of the styles are based on the belief that the body has an energy field maintained by normal breathing. Qigong unblocks stagnant qi or life force and restores normal energy flow through the body's meridians. Tai Chi is one category of QiGong.

In China and around the world, millions of people regularly practice QiGong for their health. Sessions may vary, but 20 minutes is common in many forms. The gentle, rhythmic movements are reported to reduce stress, build stamina, increase vitality, enhance the body's immune system and improve cardiovascular and respiratory functions. The slow movements activate the body's proprioception system, the sense that indicates whether the body is moving with required effort, as well as where the various parts of the body are located in relation to each other. Visualizations are used to enhance the mind-body connection to promote healing. It's practiced by all ages because its slow gentle movements can be adapted for even for the most physically challenged.

Historically it was practiced extensively in Taoist and Buddhist monasteries as part of their martial arts training. It's believe that traditional QiGong was based on the belief that certain body movements and mental concentration along with various breathing techniques would balance physical, metabolic and mental functions. Later these practices became standardized, often in connection with the various meditative techniques of religious practices. Over the centuries many new forms of QiGong were created and passed down.

QiGong can be learned from a book or video, or with a trained teacher. In many cases people begin to learn on their own and then develop their skills with professional training.

Tip #63: Chiropractic

If you suffer from chronic pain, there may be a problem with your spine which controls your nervous system and therefore your pain. The principle of chiropractic is that energy, especially of the nervous system, must flow freely through the spinal column for good body health. The relationship of the spine's structure and function to the health of the body is a concept that goes back thousands of years to writings in ancient Greece and China. Even Hippocrates, the Greek physician, (of the Hippocratic Oath for doctors) mentioned the importance of the spine to health.

Chiropractors practice a hands-on technique of healthcare that most people recognize for spinal manipulation or adjustment. Whether an injury is from a single event such as lifting something heavy or from a repetitive stress of poor posture, the result is physical and chemical changes that restrict the movement of the spine. Manipulation, whether manual or by a device, restores mobility. This reduces pain, muscle tightness and inflammation so the body can heal. Chiropractors often use what's called "passive muscle testing," meaning they observe the lengthening or shortening of the legs or arms in reaction to touching a specific spot to locate the area needing adjustment.

The therapy was developed by Daniel David Palmer in Davenport, Iowa in 1895. He began the Palmer School of Chiropractic in 1897 and it continues to be one of the most prominent chiropractic colleges to this day.

Chiropractic care has only recently gained a wide degree of acceptance and respectability. For years, the American Medical Association worked to discredit the profession but in 1976 Chester Wilk and four other chiropractors filed a lawsuit for restraint of trade. After 14 years of legal battles a federal court ruled against the AMA, finding that they had engaged in an illegal activity, the use of propaganda against chiropractic.

Tip #64: Surgical Intervention

If nothing you've tried works, then your doctor may recommend surgery for your chronic pain. Medications may mask the symptoms but if the doctor can't resolve the source of your pain and the medications aren't handling it, then his next option is surgery. Most people consider surgery as the absolute last, and most desperate, option for treatment only after they've tried everything else. Be warned that surgery may not solve your chronic pain, and in fact, may make it even worse. Doctors don't bring this up like they should, and many patients pay the price.

In some cases, the problem is due to injury to peripheral nerves—all of the nerves outside of your brain and spinal column. However, this is a difficult area for modern medicine and even diagnosing peripheral neuropathy is challenging and even then how it contributes to chronic pain isn't understood very well. If surgery is chosen, there are several different types depending on your situation.

Most people are familiar with surgical interventions for chronic pain when they have a joint replacement. This might be for hips, knees, even shoulders and it's called Arthroplasty.

When two bones in a joint are fused to get rid of the space or motion it's called Arthrodesis. Obviously this surgery itself can be a problem, since it decreases your ability to move the joint. Normally this is used on hands or feet but in my mother's case it was also used to fuse discs in her spine. Today there are different types of back surgery. The Diskectomy removes the herniated portion of a spinal disk. A Laminectomy removes a portion of the bone at the back of the spine to increase the amount of room for the nerves. Fusion is a more serious type of surgery because it removes the arthritic discs and permanently connects two or more bones in the spine. Even more serious is surgery to replace discs in your spine with ones made of plastic or metal.

The least invasive surgery is called Arthroscopic surgery. This is when a small camera called an arthroscope is used through a small incision to treat cartilage tears and other minor issues.

Whatever surgery you consider, please realize that it may not solve your chronic pain and it may actually increase it.

Tip #65: S.C.E.N.A.R or SKENAR

S.C.E.N.A.R. is an acronym for Self-Controlling Energy-Neuro Adaptive Regulation, which is both a therapy and the advanced medical treatment device. Russian inventor Alexander Karasev developed the technology after losing his sister to food poisoning. He based the original design on the TENS machine concept, but while the TENS masks pain, Scenar relieves the cause of the pain by using the principles of acupuncture to harness the body's own healing ability. The Russians funded development of the device because it would help solve the restrictions of weight and volume of medical equipment for space travel. Russia's version of the FDA approved it in 1986 and it is now widely used in Russian hospitals.

The original development group split into two different companies and the research went forward on two different but similar equipment lines called the 97.4 and the 500/600 Scenar series. In the late 1990s Russian-born doctor Zulia Valeyeva-Frost moved to London and obtained the exclusive rights to manufacture and sell the Scenar in the Americas and parts of the UK and Europe. In 2000, Jerry Tennant, M.D. accepted the position for training Scenar practitioners in America.

The SCENAR device is used by trained therapists to help the body reactivate its self-regulatory mechanism that's been pushed out of balance by accident, illness or disease. Areas of the skin that are connected in some way to stressed or injured tissues or organs will demonstrate abnormal electrical characteristics. The device stimulates the body's self-healing and immune systems for more rapid healing and pain relief. This self-regulation is achieved by the body's neuropeptides, sometimes called the body's pharmacy, being stimulated into action by the device with proper treatment protocols.

There are several different models on the market and the SCENAR is certified by the European Common Market's equivalent of the FDA for pain control. In the U.S., the technology is registered with the FDA as a biofeedback device for muscle re-education and relaxation training.

Tip #66: Nerve Blocks

I'm sure every woman has heard of epidural nerve blocks for childbirth. Many swear by its wonderful pain relief. These types of anesthetics work by preventing nerve cells from sending or relaying the coded pain electrical signals. Also called neural blockades they can be used to treat back and neck pain along with other types of chronic and acute pain.

There are different types of nerve blocks. Doctors may use a nerve block to find out what's causing your pain and where it's coming from. They can judge how you react to a temporary nerve block to better figure out the reason for your pain and how best to treat it. These are therapeutic and diagnostic nerve blocks. There are also anesthetic nerve blocks that can be applied to a wide range of nerves in the body.

A nerve block is an injection of a medication close to a targeted nerve to provide pain relief that may last a few days, weeks, or even years. These injections often are anti-inflammatory medications along with a local anesthetic. Pain relief varies from person to person and while some folks get relief from a single injection others require multiple treatments. Unfortunately some people don't experience any pain relief.

You may not be a good candidate for a nerve block if you already have an infection at the site of the injection, are on anticoagulants or have a bleeding disorder.

There are also permanent nerve blocks done with surgery that damages or destroys specific nerves. This type of surgery is reserved for the most serious cases of chronic, debilitating pain. There are different types of surgical procedures including a Sympathetic Blockade where a drug is used to block the pain by permanently destroying the nerve. There is also a Neurectomy where the doctor will remove all or part of a peripheral nerve to block it. Another type of surgical nerve block is a Rhizotomy where the root of a nerve coming from the spine is destroyed.

Tip #67: Implanted Spinal Cord Stimulation

You may remember the section about the TENS unit and how its sticky pads can be placed anywhere on your body to provide variable electrical stimulation to confuse your pain nerve signals and reduce your pain. It's frequently used to control lower back pain. There is a more serious type of device called a neurostimulator that can actually be implanted into your lower back, called a Spinal Cord Stimulation device or dorsal column stimulator. It can deliver a higher dose of pain relief, because it sends electrical pulses directly into your spine. More than 30,000 people a year undergo this type of surgery.

The SCS is a small, pacemaker type battery pack placed under the skin near your butt, combined with thin wires that are inserted between the spinal cord and the vertebrae. This is used with a remote control outside the body so you can control the amount of stimulation, which is usually felt as a light tingling sensation. If that is uncomfortable, there are newer devices that offer stimulation that can't be felt at all. Since the conventional pulse generator uses a battery, it will run out, requiring another surgery to replace it. There are also rechargeable units that work in a similar manner but don't use batteries that need to be replaced.

If this is of interest to you because drugs aren't getting the pain-control job done, or you want to reduce the amount of opioids you're taking, you'll first get a trial procedure and you'll wear a temporary device on your belt. If you're able to obtain at least a 50% reduction in pain then you'll be able to have a real device implanted. Today there are several different types of neuro-stimulators on the market including devices from Medtronic, Nevro HFX and Boston Scientific.

Complementary and Alternative Medicine

Tip #68: Sound Therapy

There is a wide variety of sound therapies, some of which have been used for hundreds of years. The range of frequencies utilized covers everything from low harmonic tones from a crystal bowl all the way up to ultrasound technology. The biological effects depend on the frequency of the sound waves. It can promote tissue healing, and treat pain.

Sound is normally associated with music and it has been used to reconnect parts of the brain so it can release the repetitive chronic pain signals. In fact, sound is an easy and direct way to stimulate the brain.

There is also Sound Wave Therapy, also called Shockwave Therapy and Extracorporeal Shockwave Therapy (ESWT), which uses high-frequency acoustic waves to target areas of the body experiencing chronic pain. This non-invasive treatment has been used for over thirty years but is gaining wider acceptance as an alternative to surgery and medications.

Diathermy Trusted Source is a treatment that creates heat beneath the skin. This type of sound wave energy is absorbed by the body, resulting in molecular vibration, which is converted into heat. In a similar matter, Cavitation Therapy uses sound waves to change the pressure in certain tissue fluids, causing bubbles to form and then burst.

You've probably heard of an ultrasound, because it can be an imaging tool to see inside the body, but it can also be used to treat pain. A 2020 clinical trial found that continuous, low-intensity ultrasound resulted in significant pain reduction for people with musculoskeletal pain in the shoulder, neck and knees. However, the FDA warns that ultrasonic therapy is not safe for everyone and says that you should talk with your doctor if you have a cardiac pacemaker, a malignancy in the target area, a healing fracture, an implanted medical device or are pregnant.

Tip #69: Deep Oscillation

This therapy uses intermittent electrostatic impulses created by a Hivamat machine for treating chronic pain. It uses friction and attraction to produce vibrations of up to 250 times per second which can have deep, relaxing effect on muscles, blood and lymph vessels, fatty tissue, skin and other conductive tissue.

The treatment is done by having the patient hold a titanium contact between their fingers or toes and then having the gloved hands of the therapist glide over the painful tissues in a circular pattern with a hand applicator that's a second contact. This has an effect going down 8 cm with no pressure. Treatment usually lasts about 30 minutes.

Tip #70: Pulsed Electro Magnetic Field (PEMF)

PEMF devices, also known as low field magnetic stimulation (LFMS), consist of a therapy mat for the patient to lie on, with an applicator to be placed against a part of the body in pain. An electric current is then sent through the copper coils in the PEMF device to generate a magnetic field that enters the body. Different physical conditions respond differently to various levels of intensity, waveforms and frequencies.

This is not the same as a TENS unit, which uses electric currents to relieve pain by blocking the pain signals. The electric currents produced by PEMF electromagnetic fields do not enter the body.

There is growing evidence that PEMF has clinically significant effects on pain, especially in patients with osteoarthritis, but there is no single PEMF device that can be used to treat everything. Also, while the FDA has approved PEMF treatments, many companies do not want to spend the time and money getting their device approved. In other words, there are a lot of scam devices on the market making lots of promises that are simply lies. For example, some PEMF devices claim to use "earth frequencies" that are supposed to be better for the body.

PEMF treatments vary depending on what is being treated, ranging from just a few minutes up to 12 hours but eight minutes is a common treatment time. While PEMF therapy is generally considered safe, people with a pacemaker or any other type of electrical implant should not use it.

Tip #71: H-Wave

The H-Wave device provides electrical stimulation to manage chronic pain, speed recovery and function. Unlike TENS and other electrical therapy devices, it is a rehabilitative device that is designed to provide pain relief after the device is turned off. The device generates a mild current that generates a non-fatiguing muscle contraction which increases blood circulation and oxygenation, which in turn promotes new blood vessel growth.

You can buy a H-Wave device over the counter to use at home on a regular basis several times a day. Treatments usually last 30 to 60 minutes but can be done while sitting in your favorite easy chair. Each device comes with personalized instruction. There are two settings. The low-frequency mode contracts muscles to accelerate recovery by helping the body get rid of congestion and waste. The high-frequency setting is designed to manage chronic pain by shutting down the nerve's pain signals.

There are studies that show these biphasic waveforms positively affect nerve function, blood and lymph flow, causing significant benefits for diabetic and non-specific neuropathic pain, improve muscle function and reduce the amount of pain medication.

Tip #72: Feldenkrais Method®

The Feldenkrais Method® is a process of educating the body, which expands the assortment of movements, enhances awareness, improves function and enables people to express themselves more fully. It is very popular with dancers, musicians and artists. It can be used by anyone who wants to reconnect with their natural ability to move, think and feel. It is also effective at improving movement-related pain and functioning in cases of stroke or cerebral palsy. It is not a massage, bodywork or necessarily a therapeutic technique, but rather a learning process. In contrast to other structural integration therapies, the Feldenkrais Method® does not adhere to an idealized form but relies on the internal wisdom of the body to find what is right.

A core belief of the Feldenkrais Method® is that improving the ability to move can improve one's overall wellbeing. It is based on principles of physics, biomechanics and an empirical understanding of learning and human development. The Method is an educational system that uses movement and awareness as the primary method for learning and its purpose is to give greater functional awareness, defined as the interaction of the person with the outside world or the self with the environment. By teaching people how their whole body cooperates in any movement helps them live their lives more fully, efficiently and comfortably.

The Feldenkrais Method® is expressed in two parallel forms. Awareness Through Movement® lessons are organized around a particular function and normally last 30-60 minutes. There are hundreds of hours of these verbally-directed movement sequences which evolve from comfortable, easy movements into movements of greater range and complexity. Functional Integration® is a hands-on form of tactile, kinesthetic communication. The practitioner communicates to the student how they organize their body by gentle touching and movement, which shows how to move in more expanded and functional ways. The lesson is usually performed lying on a table designed specifically for the work but it can also be done with the student in sitting or standing positions.

Moshe Pinhas Feldenkrais moved to Tel Aviv in 1954 and made his living for the first time solely by teaching his Functional Integration method. In the late 1950s Feldenkrais presented his work in Europe and The United States. In the mid-1960s he published *Mind and Body and Bodily Expression*. In 1967, he published *Improving the Ability to Perform*, titled *Awareness through Movement* in its 1972 English language edition.

Tip #73: Pilates

Pilates is a physical education program developed by Joseph Hubertus Pilates in the early part of the twentieth century. It is a set of principles and full-body, sequential exercises that works the whole body in balance, coordinating the upper and lower parts of the body with its center or core. It can also be used to reduce and control pain by properly aligning the body.

Born in Germany in 1880, Pilates was a frail child but grew up to become an accomplished athlete, gymnast and boxer. During World War I he was held in detention camps in England where he became a nurse and devised exercises for immobilized patients. He opened the first Pilates Studio in New York City in 1926. His first book was *Your Health* published in 1932, followed by *Return To Life Through Contrology* in 1945.

Originally called Contrology, it focuses on the core postural muscles that help keep the body balanced and provide support for the spine. Pilates exercises teach awareness of breath and alignment of the spine. Programs are uniquely tailored to each individual, which is why it can be used to treat health problems. It is very popular with dancers and performers because it builds strength and flexibility without bulk. It became known as the Pilates Method after the death of Joseph Pilates in 1967.

Pilates exercises demand complete, intense focus because they teach body awareness. This is a series of precision movements that engage both body and mind. The eight original principles of Pilates are: Concentration, Control, Centering, Flow, Precision, Breath, Relaxation and Stamina. The initial Pilates program contained 34 floor exercises but Joseph Pilates also invented several pieces of equipment with their own series of exercises. He developed the concept of the first one while serving in a detention camp in England. Using the springs from his bed he created the forerunner of the Reformer apparatus although some sources claim it was the best.

There are a variety of Pilates certifications available, so consumers are cautioned to research the training of their instructor because it is key to their ability to customize the program. Two of the main Pilates organizations are the United States Pilates Association and the Pilates Method Alliance.

Tip #74: Applied Kinesiology

Applied Kinesiology (AK) is a technique using muscle testing as a diagnostic tool and for stimulating the body's natural healing ability, an obvious goal when treating chronic pain. Today, there are an estimated 130 variations on this fundamental concept with new adaptations frequently being developed by practitioners. This process is not the same as Kinesiology which is the study of movement or physical activity, although many people confuse the terms.

In simple terms, AK uses muscle testing all over the body with no verbal questions and focuses on the structural and nutritional aspects of the body. It also uses gait analysis, range of motion evaluation and other techniques. Many chiropractors, naturopaths, medical doctors, dentists, massage therapists and acupuncturists use the process. Unfortunately the therapy is also used by others interested only in selling supplements and some less-than-reputable healing therapies. Most of the energy or specialized forms of AK use muscle testing as a biofeedback process with only straight-arm (deltoid) muscle tests while asking "yes/no" questions. These practitioners are more concerned about the mental/emotional aspects of the individual.

Although muscle testing had been recognized as far back as the 1920s in the U.S., it wasn't until Dr. George Goodheart made his presentation to an American Chiropractic Association meeting in Denver in 1964 that the term "applied kinesiology" became established. His original observation was that a weak muscle could be treated and the strength immediately improved. At first, his work focused on using muscle testing to improve chiropractic adjustments, but sometimes these treatments were not completely successful so he expanded the diagnostic and treatment options.

He noticed specific relationships between muscles and the energy meridians of Chinese medicine. Weak muscle testing would become strong when a patient touched that part of the body where the dysfunction originated, a process he called therapy localization. The process began to use the body's energy system for rapid healing. From these basic concepts, Applied Kinesiology has grown into a broad field of alternative healing. *Time* magazine named Dr. Goodheart an Alternative Medicine Innovator for his work.

The International College of Applied Kinesiology (ICAK) was founded in the 1970s and it offers training and certification by its board. Other types of applied kinesiology normally offer their own training and certification programs.

Tip #75: Healing Touch

Healing Touch is a nurturing energy therapy based on the belief that everyone has the capacity to heal through touch and compassionate intent. The technique can be used for all ages and conditions of health or illness, regardless of the type or severity of pain. It can even be used for animals.

By assisting in the balance of your physical, emotional and spiritual wellbeing, Healing Touch works with the body's energy field to support your natural ability to heal. The process uses light touch to balance and strengthen the energy field. Research has shown the process effective in improving relaxation, improving the patient's sense of wellbeing, decreasing pain, reducing side-effects of cancer treatments and providing a feeling of a positive change in energy.

The process was developed by Janet Mentgen, R.N. in Colorado during the 1980s. As a nurse she founded Healing Touch in 1989 as a program of continuing education for nursing professionals and lay people interested in healing. Today it is used in hospitals, hospices, spas and a variety of settings. She was honored in 1988 as the

holistic nurse of the year by the American Holistic Nurses'
Association (AHNA) for her work.

Healing Touch became a certificate program of the AHNA in
1990 and was then transferred to Healing Touch International, Inc.
which was created in 1995 to certify Healing Touch Practitioners
and Instructors and to promote Healing Touch worldwide. The
Healing Touch Certificate Program progresses from beginner to
advanced practitioner level using a variety of hands-on techniques
through five levels of education.

Tip #76: Hellerwork Structural Integration

Hellerwork Structural Integration combines deep-tissue structural
bodywork, movement education, and dialogue to restore the body's
natural balance. It's based on the concept that the body, mind and
spirit are inseparable so they must be treated as a whole. Only by
treating the whole body can it be restored to its natural and pain-
free condition.

Therapy is customized to each individual but built on a standard
11-step series. Most of the work done in the one-hour sessions takes
place on a massage table but sitting or standing work may also be
included. The process first works with the connective tissue to
realign the muscle-skeleton system, so restoring balance and ease of
motion. Movement education trains the person to move with
minimum effort. The dialogue process explores how thoughts,
beliefs and attitudes impact the body. Hellerwork feels like slow
deep pressure that is followed by a sensation of release. Clients may
need to make slow motions while the practitioner guides the tissue.
Practitioners are trained in the amount of pressure to use, speed and
technique but sensations may vary from pleasure to mild, temporary
discomfort based on the condition of the tissue.

Hellerwork believes that everyone is innately healthy but to
maximize your health you must develop deeper experience with
your movement, the integrity of your body and your relationship
with yourself and your world.

Joseph Heller was born in Poland in 1940 but came to the U.S. at age 16. He studied with Ida Rolf, the originator of Rolf Structural Integration, becoming a Rolfer in 1972. He also studied Structural Patterning from Judith Ashton. He became the first president of the Rolf Institute in 1975 and continued studying with Ida Rolf until 1978 when he left the Institute to create a new type of bodywork called Hellerwork.

Training and certification is done by the American Hellerwork Structural Integration Association. As a type of bodywork it requires massage licensing in most states. Please check the training, qualifications and licensing of your practitioner before beginning any type of bodywork therapy.

Tip #77: Bonnie Prudden Myotherapy

In 1976, Bonnie Prudden developed her **Myotherapy** method to relax muscle spasms, relieve pain and improve circulation. The technique is based on the concepts of trigger point injection therapy and therapeutic exercise. The term comes from "myo" for muscle and "therapy" for treatment.

"Trigger points" can begin in a muscle whenever it is damaged and are activated by either emotional or physical stress causing the muscle to spasm with pain. The basic formula is:

Trigger Points + Stress + Triggering Mechanism = Chronic Pain.

Older people often suffer from collecting more trigger points throughout their lives. Bonnie says it's pain that ages us, not years, and pain comes from someplace, usually trigger points. Fibromyalgia is a type of muscle pain that can be helped by this therapy.

Myotherapists defuse the pain by pressing or pinching on the appropriate trigger point for several seconds with fingers, knuckles or even elbows and then passively stretching the muscle into its normal relaxed and painless condition. Usually the pressing lasts less than seven seconds at each spot. Patients wear loose clothing and no shoes for a myotherapy session. The exercises taught to each patient afterwards are necessary for them to remain pain-free. Normally, patients require less than ten sessions for relief and they'll have the knowledge of how to use the therapy on themselves using tools like the Bodo and the Shepherd's Crook. The technique can even be used on animals.

Bonnie Prudden's Myotherapy® method is taught in person and through her many books, videos and media appearances. Her work on physical fitness began with her research on American school children in the 1950s, which she reported to President Dwight Eisenhower. As a result of her efforts, the federal government established the first requirements for children's fitness programs. She received the President's Council Lifetime Achievement Award in 2007.

Tip #78: Rolfing Structural Integration

Rolfing® Structural Integration was created in the 1950s by Dr. Ida Pauline Rolf as a holistic system of soft tissue manipulation and movement education. It's a unique blend of function and structure enabling the body to work in proper alignment with gravity. Chronic pain can be reduced and even eliminated by improving the alignment and functioning of the body.

Ida Rolf received her Ph.D. in biochemistry in 1920. As a result of her own and others' health issues, she researched the problems of bones, muscles and movement. One of her popular quotes is, "Some individuals may perceive their losing fight with gravity as a sharp pain in their back, others as the unflattering contour of their body, others as constant fatigue...They are off balance. They are at war with gravity."

Her study of Hatha Yoga influenced the development of Rolfing. She recognized that bodies properly aligned and functioning with gravity have less stress and pain with more energy, improved posture and body awareness. The legs are aligned to the hips, shoulders and rib cage with the body positioned correctly over the feet so that all of the joints are integrated to each other.

Rolfing begins with the Ten Series, a basic sequence of ten one-hour sessions with the patient lying down on a massage table. At times the client will be asked to walk back and forth to evaluate progress. Each session has a specific goal in the sequence. While the client is guided through each movement, the Rolfer manipulates the fascia to restore it to its original length, applying slow-moving pressure with their knuckles, thumbs, fingers, elbows and even knees. Working with the deep myofascial structures to separate layers and align muscles, the process acquired a reputation for being painful in the 1960s. Today most Rolfers work closely with clients for comfort and effectiveness since the goal is to relieve pain, not cause it.

Many clients choose a tune-up series after the initial sessions. There is also an Advanced Series of five sessions available. Today, many Rolfers also offer movement training to complement the structural integration.

In 1989, a group of dedicated followers started the Guild for Structural Integration to maintain Ida Rolf's traditional work and "the Recipe." This group of educators and practitioners has its own training programs and certification standards for GSI practitioners.

The Rolf Institute of Structural Integration (RISI) is another organization that trains and certifies Rolfers and Rolf Movement Practitioners around the world. Practitioners in the U.S. must be licensed as massage therapists, so please check your state agencies for requirements.

Tip #79: Massage

If you've ever had a massage, you know how relaxing it can be and how it can loosen up muscles that have been tightened by pain. A massage is the process of applying pressure, tension, motion, or vibration to the soft tissues of the body. Working on the muscles, tendons, ligaments, joints, connective tissue or lymph system for a positive response can be done manually or with the aid of a device. In addition to just feeling wonderful, it can be a form of therapy for all or part of the body, to help injuries heal, relieve stress, improve circulation or to help control pain. It is one of the oldest forms of therapy, having been used by a variety of cultures for thousands of years.

There are many different types of massage to choose from but there are several basic principles. First, good communication is essential to a beneficial massage. Client and massage therapist need to talk about what's expected before beginning the session. What areas need work or need to be avoided? How much pressure is comfortable? In addition, the client's medical history and current physical condition need to be reviewed, especially if getting a massage for pain relief.

Depending on the type, massage can involve the client lying on a massage table, sitting in a massage chair, or lying on a pad on the floor. In the U.S., clients are usually unclothed but draped with towels or sheet for warmth and privacy. The massage may be done beginning with the client facing up or down and then reversing for the second half of the session.

Please note that the American Massage Therapy Association began the National Certification Exam in 1992. This exam is often used by states to regulate massage practitioners. Please check with your state's certification agency regarding local laws and regulations for massage therapists. Always remember to ask about your massage therapist's training and experience before beginning a massage.

A partial list of the types of available massage includes:

- Barefoot Deep Tissue
- Chair Massage or Corporate Massage
- Deep Tissue Massage
- Foot Massage
- Graston Technique®
- Indian Head Massage
- Lomilomi Massage
- Muscle Energy Technique (MET)
- Myofascial Release
- Neuromuscular Massage

- Petrissage Massage
- Russian Clinical Massage
- Shiatsu
- Sports Massage
- Stone Massage
- Swedish Massage
- Thai massage and
- Tui na.

For more information on these types of massage and more please read my book *How To UnBreak Your Health*.

Tip #80: Yoga

In the U.S., yoga is considered mainly a form of exercise concentrating on postures (asanas) and breathing. The rest of the world recognizes yoga as a means for both physical health and spiritual mastery. Yoga connects the movement of the body with the rhythm of the breath and the mind, which can do wonders to control chronic pain.

Yoga is a collection of ancient spiritual practices originating in India for integrating mind, body and spirit to achieve oneness with the universe. While it is one of the schools of Hindu philosophy, it is a spiritual practice, not a religion, and it does not require any specific beliefs for participation. Yoga is also central to Buddhism, Tibetan Buddhism, Jainism, and has influenced many other religions.

A male who practices yoga is a yogi, and a female practitioner is a yogini. While there is a lot of crossover between yoga schools and variations within each style, there are many common features. Hatha yoga is the most popular style in the U.S. It was introduced in the 15th century as an outgrowth of an older style known as Raja yoga. It is used to prepare the body for higher meditation. Because it develops health and flexibility, students in the U.S. are usually not interested in the complete Hatha yoga process, which deals with spiritual development.

Hatha represents opposing energies such as hot and cold, male and female, in a similar fashion to the Chinese concept of yin and yang. It works to balance the mind and body by physical exercises called asanas using controlled breathing, and the calming of the mind through relaxation and meditation. These postures develop balance, strength, and reduce stress.

It is important to find both a yoga style and yoga teacher you're comfortable with for the best results. The traditional instructions for Hatha yoga include having a glass of fresh water before the session. The asanas should be done on an empty stomach to prevent discomfort and are best done in the early morning. Asanas should not involve force or pressure, and movements should be slow and gentle. Breathing should always be done through the nose and in a controlled manner. Yoga should be done in a peaceful, clean, well-lit well-ventilated room.

Ananda yoga is a way to release unwanted tensions and to grow spiritually. This system uses silent affirmations while holding a posture, a technique intended to deepen and enhance the subtle benefits of each asana. This is a technique for aligning the body, its energy, and the mind with a series of gentle postures created to move energy upward to the brain.

Anusara Yoga® is said to mean, "stepping into the current of divine will." This new system developed by John Friend blends the human spirit with the science of biomechanics. It is different from other yoga systems by three features: Attitude; Alignment and Action.

Ashtanga yoga is a system of six, fast-paced series of sequential postures of increasing difficulty that get you sweating.

Bikram yoga is also called hot yoga because room temperatures can be near 100° Fahrenheit. This environment helps move toxins out of the body by sweating. There is a series of 26 traditional Hatha postures directed at each body system.

Hatha Yoga is often a blending of different styles of yoga under what has become almost a generic banner. This being the case, it's probably a good idea to check into the class to see if it's more in the meditative or active style before signing up. It might not hurt to check into the teacher's training and experience, too.

Integral Yoga is the form of yoga Sri Swami Satchidananda developed in 1966 to help people integrate the teachings of yoga into their everyday life. This is to promote greater peace and tolerance in the individual.

Integrative Yoga Therapy was introduced in 1993 in San Francisco by Joseph Le Page, M.A. This is a yoga teacher-training program designed specifically for medical environments such as hospitals and rehabilitation centers.

Iyengar Yoga puts an intense focus on the subtleties of each position by requiring students to hold each position longer. Students can pay close attention to the precise muscular and skeletal alignment this system demands with this longer attention. The system also uses props such as belts and chairs to deal with special needs such as injuries.

Jivamukti Yoga is a highly meditative form that is also physically challenging. Sessions may include chanting, meditation, readings, music, and affirmations along with the postures.

Kali Ray Tri Yoga® was created in 1980 as a new, flowing method of yoga. Tri Yoga fundamentals include relaxation-in-action, wave-like spinal movements and economy of motion. With the systematic approach students can remain with Basics or progress to subsequent levels. Music accompanies the classes, ending with meditation.

Kundalini Yoga was a secret process that came from the Tantra yoga path until Yogi Brahan introduced it to the West in 1969. It is supposed to help seekers of enlightenment from all religious paths tap into their greater potential. This system uses postures and dynamic breathing techniques along with chanting and meditating on mantras. Students focus on awakening the energy at the base of the spine and drawing it upward through each of the traditional seven chakras.

Phoenix Rising Yoga Therapy is a synthesis of traditional yoga and contemporary body-mind psychology that can produce a release of physical tensions and emotional blocks.

Power Yoga was a term Beryl Bender Birch created to describe Ashtanga yoga to Americans. It's a workout of a series of poses designed not to create heat and energy flow but to serve as a traditional methodology for spiritual transformation. Because of the athletic and powerful nature of the physical portion of the system, it's popular in health clubs and gyms.

Sahara Yoga is a method of meditation created in 1970 to bring a new level of awareness. The process is supposed to help you experience the power of the divine as your awareness expands. Thus, students become more integrated and balanced, capable of effortless spiritual growth.

Sivananda Yoga is a path to learn about who you really are. It is supposed to help you appreciate each level of experience.

Svaroopa® Yoga teaches different ways of doing familiar poses. It focuses on opening the spine by beginning at the tailbone and progressing through each area. This is a consciousness-oriented yoga that also promotes healing, using what many consider a very approachable style.

Tibetan Yoga is composed of five flowing movements. It is an active workout that features constant motion. Students may begin with 10 or 12 repetitions and work their way up to the 21 repetitions of the full routine.

Viniyoga is a practice designed to work on all levels. The poses are synchronized with the breath. It is a process for developing a style to meet each person's needs as they grow.

White Lotus Yoga is a flowing style that varies from gentle to vigorous depending on ability and comfort level. Classes involve alignment, breath, and the theories of yoga.

Tip #81: The Alexander Technique

Frederick Matthias Alexander (or F.M. Alexander) developed the Alexander Technique to help the body to function more efficiently due to his own medical problems. As an actor who developed chronic laryngitis resulting from his performances, he was determined to find a way to heal himself. Eventually he discovered that his problem resulted from excess muscle tension and he realized that if neck tension is reduced then the head no longer presses down on the spine, so it is free to lengthen. Many types of chronic pain have similar origins of minor issues becoming major problems.

The process of how we acquire new movements, constantly adapting and changing from our basic, primary motion can cause all sorts of health problems including chronic pain. As we grow and continually apply these changes, we grow numb to how they differ from our natural motions. Alexander called this principle the Debauchery of the Senses but scientists today label it sensory adaptation. The relationship between the neck and head was the Primary Control and the focal point of his work.

The Alexander Technique applies this principle to improve the freedom of movement for the entire body by re-education in new ways to sit, lie down, stand up and other daily functions. By learning the proper amount of energy for an activity, the body retains more energy while maintaining greater balance and coordination. The technique is about unlearning the tension the body has accumulated throughout its lifetime and the resulting muscle tension that produces abnormal mannerisms and motions, which can result in pain.

The technique is often taught to improve performance in the arts such as music, acting, dance and even in some sports training. The Julliard School of Performing Arts, the Royal College of Music and the Royal College of Dramatic Art in London are just a few of the institutions teaching this technique. It's also used as therapy to aid the recovery of balance and motion, and for speech training to repair the voice. It's even been used to unlearn repetitive stress and to aid those patients dealing with reduced mobility such as those with Parkinson's disease. Today many professional athletes are beginning to learn this technique because they also want to maximize performance with minimum wear and tear on their body. People of all ages have used the Alexander Technique to improve the quality of their lives for over a century. Training in this self-healing technique is done both in group and individual lessons.

Teachers certified by professional societies are often required to complete a 3-year program consisting of more than 1,500 hours of training. Some teachers are trained by an informal, apprentice process. Membership in professional organizations is a matter of personal choice so it is best to learn about any potential Alexander Technique teacher's training prior to beginning any therapy.

Tip #82: Naprapathy

Naprapathy was introduced in the U.S. by Dr. Oakley Smith in 1907 as a treatment process for evaluating and healing damaged connective tissues. The term comes from the Czech word "naprapravit" meaning "to connect" and the Greek word "pathos" for "suffering." This treatment technique for structural imbalances deals with sources of pain that can become chronic. This pain often begins in the spine and spreads throughout the body, causing locomotor disorders. His discovery of this therapy was the result of his own lifelong search for better health, after he had already tried chiropractic care and osteopathy. He found that this new system used bones as levers with a gentle motion and was a different type of therapy.

Poor posture, trauma from sports injuries or whiplash, and even general wear can be the cause of the imbalances causing the deterioration of the suppleness in connective tissues like ligaments. Such inelastic tissues produce stiffness, which can progress to cause pinched nerves, contributing to health problems like arthritis, carpal tunnel syndrome, Temporomandibular Joint (TMJ) Syndrome and other aches and pains.

The primary method of treatment by Doctors of Naprapathy (DN) is manipulation of the spine, focusing on the underlying ligaments along with the joints and soft tissues. Practitioners of Naprapathy, or Naprapaths, can also use ultrasound, electrical pain relief treatments along with heat and cold therapies and even lasers. To assist treatments, they may also use back braces, neckbands, taping and various types of joint supports along with posture and dietary counseling. Patients learn to appreciate their responsibility for their own health with a goal of decreasing dependence on therapy.

The National College of Naprapathic Medicine in Chicago is the original school of Naprapathy and it remains the only one offering programs to receive a DN or Doctor of Naprapathy degree. Naprapaths are licensed in Illinois and New Mexico, regulated in Ohio and may practice in other states that offer freedom of access statutes.

Tip #83: Breathwork

Breathwork uses the power of our breathing to help control pain. Women use it when they're giving birth. Athletes often force themselves to use it to control the pain of an injury. From slow, rhythmic breathing to fast panting, there are many differences in the speed and depth of our breath and they all have different effects on our pain levels.

Breathwork or conscious breathing also has many different techniques under a variety of names. Rebirthing, also called Rebirthing Breathwork, is a special breathing technique based on the concept that breathing energy along with air has therapeutic effects on the body. The increase of physical and spiritual energy has a cleansing effect on the body.

Breathwork is also a vital component of Mindfulness.

Tip #84: Craniosacral Therapy

Also known as Cranial Osteopathy and Craniopathy, Craniosacral Therapy or CST is based on the belief that all living tissues have a motion of life, which produces rhythmic impulses. Up to this point doctors studied the human skull by examining corpses, but an unusual accident offered one doctor the chance to study a living skull. This "Breath of Life" was discovered by osteopath Dr. William Sutherland more than 100 years ago. He realized that cranial bones were designed to provide a small amount of motion, which he compared to the motion of gills on a fish. These movements involve a network of tissues and fluids at the core of the human body such as spinal fluid, fluid surrounding the brain and the central nervous system. The ability of cells and tissues to express this primary motion is a vital feature for determining our general health.

There are at least three different rhythms in this "primary respiratory system," each with its own rate of vibration and pulse. These pulses are identified as: the cranial rhythmic impulse, the mid-tide, and the long tide. Practitioners feel or "listen" through their hands to the patient's body rhythms to detect any patterns of congestion or restriction. They then apply gentle pressure to improve the functioning of the central nervous system so the body can better heal itself from a wide variety of health issues, even the dizziness from a concussion.

Manipulation of the skull has actually been practiced for thousands of years, going back to Egypt, India and Peru. Dr. Sutherland began to teach his therapeutic techniques to remove restrictions in this motion to other osteopaths in the 1930s. It is referred to as craniosacral osteopathy and it is still taught today. Restoring the natural motions to the body relieves pain and allows the body to better heal itself.

The most common form of craniosacral therapy was developed in the 1970s by Dr. John E. Upledger. His technique resulted from his research at Michigan State University and he began teaching his full-body form of therapy to non-osteopaths, making it much more widely available. By 2009 the Upledger Institute had taught more than 100,000 practitioners in more than fifty countries around the world.

SomatoEmotional Release is a process developed by John Upledger that expands on the concepts of his CST. It's a process that helps to rid the mind and body of residual effects of a past trauma. "Soma" is Greek for "body," so it can be seen as psychotherapy for the body's memories. Such emotional trauma stored in the body can inhibit structural release so it is a complementary technique to CST.

Craniopathy began as chiropractic craniopathy in the 1920s by M.B. Dejarnette, D.C., D.O. as Sacro Occipital Technique. By 1968 he felt his system was sufficiently developed and began teaching craniopathy to the chiropractic profession.

A newer variation based on cranial osteopathy is Biodynamic Craniosacral Therapy. This style takes a whole-person approach to healing and the inter-connections of mind, body and spirit.

There is also a type of massage referred to as craniosacral, so it's best to check the training and qualifications of your therapist. You could be getting simply a head massage instead of therapy. In the U.S., the process has a variety of licensing requirements, so check your local regulations.

Tip #85: Magnetic Therapy

Magnetic Therapy or Magnet Therapy or Magnotherapy has been around for more than 2,000 years in a variety of civilizations as a method for natural healing and pain relief. It makes use of the static magnetic fields produced by permanent magnets in a variety of products such as bracelets, blankets, shoe insoles and other items. When combined with the reduction of stressful electromagnetic fields it's called Biomagnetic Therapy. Electromagnetic Therapy or Magnetobiology is the use of electromagnetic energy to the body for the treatment of disease.

There are two schools of thought about how this therapy functions in the human body. The first concept is biologically based, noting that there are metals like iron in our blood and cells. The use of a magnetic field on a wound or injury simply attracts the metals in our blood in order to increase the flow of oxygen, nutrients, hormones and other healing factors to that location.

The other concept is based on energy medicine and the belief of a life force in the human body that's been called Chi in Traditional Chinese Medicine or Prana in Ayurvedic medicine. It is considered a force of nature similar in some ways to gravity. Illness, injury, disease and even pain produce interruptions in the natural flow of this living energy and the use of magnets helps to restore the natural balance of this flow. It is believed that our bodies produce negative energy as a normal healing response, so a negative pole is frequently used.

Magnetic devices are now registered as medical devices available by prescription in 54 countries around the world, while the Food and Drug Administration classifies the application of magnetic fields as "not essentially harmful."

Tip #86: Reiki

Reiki (pronounced ray-key) is a style of Japanese energy work, a technique for stress reduction and relaxation to promote healing and relieve chronic pain. The term is composed of two Japanese words, "rei" meaning God's wisdom or power and "ki" meaning life force or energy.

As with other types of energy work, this process is done by moving and waving hands slightly above the individual's body in order to manipulate their ki, or life force energy. Some practitioners use a very light touch. Traditional practitioners usually hold each hand position for several minutes before moving to the next location but there are variations in technique. If an individual's energy is low, blocked or hindered in any way due to chronic pain, they are more likely to feel stress and become even more ill. Higher energy levels produce health and feelings of wellness. Moving the hands allows the Reiki practitioner to add, move and adjust this living energy. Reiki also uses symbols to attract healing energy during the process.

The ability to perform Reiki is transferred to the student during an "attunement" process by a Reiki master. This allows a Reiki student to tap into the unlimited supply of life force energy to improve their health and the health of others.

There are different types of Reiki. The original form was created by Dr. Mikao Usui in Japan during his Isyu Guo training when Reiki energy entered his crown chakra enhancing his healing abilities. Following this experience, he could give healing to others without depleting his own life force energy. Many years later he added the Reiki Ideals to add spiritual balance to Usui Reiki. For the process to have lasting results, the client must accept responsibility for her or his healing and take an active part in it.

Dr. Chujiro Hayashi received his Reiki Master initiation from Dr. Usui and he went on to open a Reiki clinic in Toyko. He developed the standard hand positions, the system of three degrees and other additions to the Reiki process.

Reiki was considered Japanese, meant only for Japanese, but Mrs. Hawayo Takata from Hawaii was so insistent on learning it after the process cured her that Dr. Hayashi relented and agreed to train her. She returned home in 1937 to introduce Reiki to the West. In 1938 Dr. Hayashi initiated her as his thirteenth and final Reiki Master.

Karuna Reiki is another type. Karuna is a Sanskrit word meaning taking action to diminish the pain and suffering of others. It's used both in Hinduism and Buddhism. There are four Karuna® symbols used in this version of Reiki.

Raku Kai Reiki was developed by Arthur Robertson, a student of one of Mrs. Takata's Reiki Masters. The technique incorporates the Tibetan practices of the Hui Yin, the Breath of the Fire Dragon, along with Tibetan symbols. This style is believed to have influenced the creation of Vajra Reiki, Tera Mai Reiki and other forms.

Reiki training was added to the curriculum of the Center for Spiritual Development in 1989 and in 1991 the name was changed to The Center for Reiki Training. Training is available in a variety of styles including the Usui/Hayashi method as taught by Mrs. Takata, combined with a style based on Tibetan shamanism called Raku Kai and traditional Japanese Reiki techniques.

There are many different levels of training and proficiency of Reiki instructors and practitioners. Before you begin your healing process with Reiki, the very first question you should ask is "What is my lineage?" because that's one of the first lessons learned in traditional training. If the practitioner has learned "microwave Reiki" or Americanized Reiki, they won't be able to answer the question and you should leave immediately and find another practitioner.

Tip #87: Advanced Jaffe-Mellor Technique™ (JMT)

JMT™ is the abbreviation for Jaffe-Mellor Technique, developed by founders Carolyn Jaffe, Doctor of Acupuncture and Ph.D. candidate in Naturopathy, and Judith Mellor, RN, Ph.D. candidate in Nutrition and certified Chinese medical herbalist. Their combined experience includes various types of acupuncture, herbology and a variety of healing processes.

This is a bioenergetic therapy that uses muscle resistance testing (MRT), a form of applied kinesiology, as the diagnostic tool to identify the pathogenic microorganisms they believe are the cause of many autoimmune diseases. The process may be beneficial for conditions such as osteoarthritis, rheumatoid arthritis, lupus, fibromyalgia, chronic fatigue syndrome, interstitial cystitis, Crohn's disease, colitis, Lyme disease, scleroderma and Multiple Sclerosis. The technique created by Jaffe and Mellor is unique in the way it employs blind testing and focused specific questions to the patient. The original process used vials of materials in the testing process but it has evolved to the point that vials are no longer used, hence the new designation, "advanced."

During the examination, the practitioner views changes in the strength of an isolated muscle against an established baseline. Arm muscles are normally used but any muscle can be tested. MRT is valuable as a diagnostic tool because it functions on a subconscious level where the autonomic nervous system resides, the system controlling all bodily functions. In other words, the process looks around behind the conscious mind to see what's happening inside.

Treatment is a gentle tapping of back muscles with either an activator (a chiropractic adjusting instrument) or an arthrostim, a device that provides mild percussion in rapid succession. The technique elicits the proper sensory input to produce more control of body function by the nervous system. The JMT™ protocol allows for as many as ten corrections during any one visit, but the actual number of corrections varies by condition. Practitioners may dispense homeopathic remedies on a temporary basis to help the body eliminate toxic materials that have built up in the tissues as a result of the disease process.

Tip #88: Energy Medicine

The new science of Energy Medicine or Electrotherapy is based on the scientific discovery of a new circulatory system in the human body for electrical energy. This process is remarkably similar to the meridian concepts of Traditional Chinese Medicine.

This new perspective on energy in the human body was developed by internationally renowned Swedish radiologist and surgeon, Dr. Bjorn E. W. Nordenstrom and published in *Biologically Closed Electrical Circuits* (1983). Beginning in the mid-1950s, Dr. Nordenstrom noticed radiating patterns around cancer tumors on chest X-rays, which he called corona structures because they reminded him of the sun's corona. Additional study revealed fluctuating electrical charges within the tumors. This led to the discovery of a new type of system, an electrical circuit that involves the transportation of ions and electrons throughout the body. This circulating current helps maintain the body's equilibrium and healing processes by influencing cellular structure and function.

Blood plasma and interstitial fluid are examples of media capable of conducting current while blood vessel walls, cells and membranes surrounding interstitial spaces provide insulation to the surroundings. In other words, they're insulated electric cables providing communication within the body through electromagnetic signaling. These flowing electrical charges found in the body resemble the "yin and yang" concepts and the flow of Chi discovered 5,000 years ago in ancient China.

The editor of The American Institute of Stress, Paul J. Rosch, M.D., F.A.C.P., wrote in his review of the 1983 book that "…he has demonstrated how specific DC microcurrents that restore ion electricity balance can be utilized to treat metastic lung cancer and other malignancies with amazing success, and his therapeutic triumphs have now been replicated by others in thousands of patients." Following a report by Dr. Tim Johnson on ABC's *20/20* program, host Barbara Walters expressed amazement at this medical breakthrough. More than 12,000 cancer patients around the world have now successfully been treated with electrochemical therapy (EChT) using Dr. Nordenstrom's BCEC concepts.

There have only been a few limited trials being conducted in America. In what may be one of the most fundamental paradigm shifts in medicine since William Harvey discovered blood circulation 350 years ago, America has taken a back seat in research. Unable to secure funding and support in America, Dr. Nordenstrom was welcomed by China to continue his research. The current five year survival rates for liver cancer are reported to be about 15% in China compared to 5% in the U.S. where they're treated with conventional therapies. In 2001, Dr. Nordenstrom received the International Scientific and Technological Cooperation Award from the People's Republic of China for his work.

EChT treatment is available in Germany, China and other countries. Costs are reported to be in the $7,500 (U.S.) range with treatment taking up to two weeks.

The fundamental premise of this new field of Electrotherapy is wound healing because it artificially enhances the body's natural healing process. The technique is being used for vision treatments and other health problems such as chronic pain.

The International Association for Biologically Closed Electric Circuits in Medicine and Biology (IABC) was founded in 1993 for the development of electrotherapeutic, thermotherapeutic and magnetotherapeutic techniques, along with conventional therapies, for the treatment of health problems including cancer.

Tip #89: Bach Flower Therapy

Many people may question why Bach Flower Therapy is listed in a book about chronic pain, but since the U.S. Pain Foundation lists it as one of their complementary therapies, it must be good enough for this book. It was also included in my earlier work *How To UnBreak Your Health*. Remember that your pain comes from your nerves, so anything that can change your nerves will help your pain.

Bach Flower Essence Therapy (also called simply FET) was created by Dr. Edward Bach to transfer the essential energy of the plant to other living organisms. This transfer causes a beneficial shift in the living energy system (chi, prana, etc.) of the person, animal or plant, empowering it to heal, which is the goal for anyone suffering from chronic pain. It's claimed that these essences (or remedies as they're called in England) can adjust the circuitry of the human nervous system altering emotional responses, replacing negative emotions with positive. It's also claimed that spiritually they open the pathway for the soul so we can fulfill our destiny. This therapy does not treat physical disease or illness directly but instead treats the emotional and mental conditions which are the source of the health problem.

This system of 38 flower essences is divided into seven groups: Fear, Uncertainty, Insufficient Interest, Loneliness, Oversensitivity, Despondency/Despair, and Over-care for Other's Welfare. Bach Flower Essences range from Agrimony to Willow and are created by infusing natural spring water with wild flowers either by the sun-steep process or simply by boiling. Each essence contains 27% grape brandy as a preservative.

Treatment can range from taking four drops four times each day, usually mixed with mineral water, to taking two drops in a glass of water sipped at regular intervals throughout the day. The frequency of dosage is more important than the quantity consumed and in severe or chronic conditions the dosage may be taken hourly. It's possible to put the drops into a hot drink, which offers the additional benefit of evaporating the alcohol. They can even be put into carbonated beverages and other drinks.

It's possible and often necessary to mix essences together to meet the unique mix of emotions causing problems, so it's not uncommon to take up to seven essences together at the same time. However, fewer elements are always considered better. It was suggested to Dr. Bach that he simply mix all of his remedies together but when he tried it, the mixture didn't work at all. Each combination can be taken for at least a month and normal treatment periods last from three to six months. Treatments should not be taken for more than a year. The only pre-mixed formula is sold under the name Rescue Remedy and it's designed specifically to treat an emergency situation or crisis.

Dr. Edward Bach was a British physician, bacteriologist and later pathologist who worked on vaccines and a set of homeopathic nosodes, which are still called the seven Bach Nosodes. The NIH defines nosodes (from the Greek *nosos*, disease) as biological preparations used in homeopathic medicine to prevent disease. He died in 1936 at the age of 50 but he had been diagnosed with cancer in 1917 and given only three months to live. He treated himself successfully for 19 years with these natural potions. During his career, he saw disease as the physical result of unhappiness, fear and worry, so in 1930 he left his London practice and moved to the country to create a new system of medicine based on nature.

It is possible to self-diagnose and select essences simply by reading one of the many books on the subject. There are also trained practitioners available for consultation. All Bach Flower Essences have a "use-by" date of five years from creation due to the shelf life of the brandy in the rubber-topped bottle, although their energy properties last indefinitely. They are available in retail stores and on the Internet. This therapy has also been used to calm hyperactive dogs, fearful cats and other problem pet emotions.

Tip #90: Aromatherapy

As long as we're talking about flowers and smell, let's move on to Aromatherapy. This is the ancient concept of using potent distilled extracts of flowers, fruits, grasses, leaves, spices, roots, woods and other organic substances to stimulate the organs, the healing systems of the body and to enhance psychological wellbeing. As a holistic healing process, it is able to work on several different levels. Using essential oils, the approach delivers various scents to the body directly through the skin by massage or inhaled through the nose.

The use of the olfactory sense provides for an immediate response and easy absorption into the bloodstream, even when the subject has a stuffy nose and can't smell. This pathway is especially powerful because it is the only place in the body where the central nervous system is directly exposed to contact with the environment. Once an olfactory cell is activated, it sends a signal directly to the limbic part of the brain. In most cases our subconscious mind has already received and reacted to the signal due to our memories and emotions before we are consciously aware of the sensation.

Essential oils have been used for thousands of years. The Chinese may have been the first to use them along with incense to create harmony and balance. The Egyptians used different types of oils to prepare their dead for entombment, in cosmetics, as medicines, and for spiritual purposes. It wasn't until the 16th century that essential oils became available in an apothecary. In 1928, French chemist René-Maurice Gattefossé created the term aromatherapy as part of his work with essential oils. Today, aromatherapy is growing in popularity as part of the return to more natural types of healing. A few drops of essential oils can simply be put on a tissue and inhaled, or a professional atomizer may be used. Drops can also be placed on acupuncture points to boost healing or they can be used in massage. Many people are familiar with aromatherapy, hangvi used Vicks Vaporub, a product that uses eucalyptus.

Essential oils are produced by different techniques depending on the organic source, including cold-pressed, steam and the absolute distillation process. Hospitals and nursing homes in America are beginning to use Aromatherapy and clinical studies in the United Kingdom are speeding acceptance in Europe. Properly stored, essential oils may last up to seven years.

The olfactory sense was the subject of the 2004 Nobel Laureate in Physiology or Medicine recognizing that 3% of our genes create olfactory receptor cells which enable human beings to detect 10,000 different odors.

Perfume oils or fragrances are not the same as essential oils, since they contain manmade chemicals, although there are some natural perfumers. Be aware that synthetic products are available which claim to have aromatherapy properties. As with all products, holistic or not, Buyer Beware is a wise precaution.

Tip #91: Crystal Therapy

Crystal Therapy, also called Gem Therapy, has its roots in ancient cultures as diverse as Ayurveda, Chinese medicine, and Native American shamanism. It is another type of holistic therapy that focuses on the person as a whole instead of being preoccupied just with symptoms. The goal of this therapy is to restore balance and wholeness of mind, spirit and body, which will heal your chronic pain.

The basic tenets are that human beings are unique, interconnected fields of energy and blockages of our energy flow result in illness and disease. Each type of gemstone expresses a different color and frequency of energy that can be used to address different types of blockages to restore energy flow and health.

For example, according to ancient texts, Ruby can improve emotional stability such as healing from painful and suppressed emotions and is good for the heart, spleen and hypertension. Green gems like Emerald are beneficial for supporting the immune system, and Blue Sapphire can clear the mind, restore mental balance and help strengthen weak bones and nerves and increase vitality. Gemstone energy can be used on specific energy centers like the chakras or acupressure points or to treat the whole energy system. They're used to treat illnesses and to prevent health problems.

Gemstones are thought to be intense concentrations of energy because they were formed over eons often under extreme pressure. The shape of a gemstone affects its ability to express energy. The ideal shape is a sphere because it can radiate its power evenly in all directions. To be effective, stones must also have no impurities to contaminate the energy and they must be of therapeutic quality. While there are over 100 gem therapy protocols reported it is possible to obtain benefits simply by wearing therapeutic gems around the neck.

Another innovation and variation of gem therapy is Electronic Gem Therapy, which uses gemstones in lighting devices. By using colored light energy, it is possible to deliver specific energy to selected parts of the body. Lamp therapy is even being used by some veterinarians.

Crystal Healing is a variation of gem therapy that uses only natural crystals. Different colored crystals radiate different frequencies of energy that can be used for healing, for strengthening the body and resolving issues.

Crystal Bowl Therapy is another way to use crystals, this time for sound or vibration therapy to heal the body's energy system. Sound has been used for healing in many cultures around the world for thousands of years. Tibetans continue to use bells, bowls of crystal or brass along with other devices as part of their religious practices. If you've ever run a wet finger around the rim of a wine glass then you're familiar with the type of vibrations a crystal bowl can produce.

This therapy is based on the concept that everything in the universe, including our bodies, vibrates at a particular frequency of energy. Parts of your body have different frequencies, so when something is vibrating out of tune or out of harmony with the rest of the body resulting from an energy blockage, there is disease or illness. Using sound vibrations that are felt and heard, it is possible to open the blockages and correct the resonant frequency of the chakras, meridians and other energy centers. This process is designed to restore harmony between the physical and subtle or energy body.

Today crystal bowls are made from crushed quartz that is almost 100% pure, melted into molds. They come in a variety of sizes, typically 10" to 24", to produce at least the seven tones which correspond to the seven main chakra centers. They are made to "sing" by running a device like a suede-covered mallet around the edge of the bowl. Sounds from these bowls can also used in meditation, to supplement massage therapy, yoga sessions, even to complement energy therapies like Reiki.

Tip #92: Water Therapy

One type of water therapy is called Watsu® therapy, which is one of the early forms of aquatic bodywork. It combines elements of shiatsu, muscle stretching, massage and dance with graceful, fluid movements in a warm water environment. Working in water requires the client to be supported at all times, which creates a connection between therapist and client that is much deeper than work done on a table. The therapeutic benefits of warm water include greater freedom of movement and deep relaxation.

The technique was developed in 1980 by Harold Dull, a Northern California massage therapist. After returning from Japan he began floating his Zen Shiatsu students in the warm water of Harbin Hot Springs. The idea of stretching to open the flow of energy channels is even older than acupuncture. Stretching also strengthens muscles and increases flexibility. The support provided by working in warm water relieves compression in joints like vertebrae and decreases muscle tension, allowing movement that is not possible out of the water and helps to reduce pain.

In addition to traditional Watsu®, there are three major styles: Waterdance, Healing Dance, and the Jahara Technique. Waterdance is done completely beneath the surface. The Healing Dance style is a mix between regular Watsu and Waterdance. The Jahara Technique is called the gentlest form because of its constant support and gentle bodywork. One of the common features are moments of stillness alternated with rhythmical, flowing movements, often using the Water Breath Dance, which is the rising and falling back caused by each breath. Originally Watsu® involved a therapist supporting the client, but with the use of floatation devices today there is a greater range of movement possible. Sessions are usually 50-60 minutes but can vary depending on your therapist and health condition.

Watsu® is practiced in more than 40 countries and is accepted as a key methodology in rehabilitation by aquatic therapists. The Worldwide Aquatic Bodywork Association (WABA) supervises Watsu® standards along with maintaining a registry of authorized practitioners.

There is another type of water therapy known as Floatation Therapy, originally known as sensory deprivation. It was created in 1954 by Dr. John C. Lilly, an American neurophysiologist and psychoanalyst. He expected to learn about the brain in sleep states but discovered that the mind becomes even more active when deprived of outside stimulation. It's also been called Restricted Environmental Stimulation Technique (REST) since the 1970s. The process produces profound relaxation, which allows the mind and body to regenerate natural energy without interference. There are similarities between this process and some forms of meditation. This form of relaxation can help reduce chronic pain.

There are two major types of floatation devices, wet or dry. Clients float directly in the water in the wet version, but rest on a sheet of plastic on top of the water in the dry version. Most floatation tanks measure about eight feet long and four feet wide and contain just enough very warm water to float. The water is loaded with salts and minerals, making it nearly impossible to sink. Clients will shower before and after each session, which may last from one to two hours. There are variations depending on customer preferences such as complete darkness or having a little light, and having the tank completely closed or with the lid slightly left open. Some people prefer total quiet while others request soft music or even self-hypnosis tapes for losing weight or to stop smoking. There is usually a 2-way microphone built into the tank for communication and safety.

The deep relaxation produced by this environment has beneficial effects on the body, primarily in increased healing capacity. There are also psychological benefits connected with the process. By reducing stress it's been useful in the treatment of obsessive and addictive behaviors. Floatation tanks may be found in health clubs and spas or even purchased for home use.

I would like to point out that there are warnings about this type of therapy if you have a history of psychological disorders, especially claustrophobia.

Tip #93: Bee Venom Therapy

Bee-Venom Therapy (BVT), also called bee-sting therapy, is one type of Apitherapy or the therapeutic use of beehive products such as honey or royal jelly. The use of bees and bee products goes back to ancient Egypt, Greece and China, but Hungarian doctor Bodog Beck popularized the treatment in the 1930s.

It's believed that bee stings work to stimulate the body's immune system in specific locations, training it to become stronger each time, a process similar to a weightlifter increasing weights at each workout. It may also increase the body's production of cortisol, which is critical to reducing pain. Bee stings are commonly thought to ease the symptoms of arthritis, MS, fibromyalgia, irritable bowel syndrome (IBS) and other conditions.

BVT may use up to 80 stings per day with live bees by urging them to sting the affected area, on trigger points or acupuncture centers. The therapy normally is used about three times per week with a gradual increase in the number of stings. The highest potency bee venom comes directly from a live bee in the late spring or early fall. Standardized bee venom solution may also be injected or can be used in a cream or ointment. Bee venom is a complex source of peptides, enzymes with at least 18 active components which have pharmaceutical properties although the exact mechanism of its function is unknown. It's also a volatile substance which may lose potency from a variety of factors.

Because about 2% of the population may have allergic reactions to bee stings, the first step is to test the risk factor by injecting a very small amount of bee venom underneath the skin or with a single bee sting. If no allergic reaction develops, the therapy continues by testing a little more venom. In any case, it is always a smart idea for anyone using BVT to have a bee sting kit with a syringe of epinephrine close at hand for safety. Even if you haven't had a problem with the first 79 stings doesn't mean you won't have a problem with the 80th. Allergic reactions can include anaphylactic shock, which can be fatal.

Bee venom has been approved by the FDA for desensitization purposes only.

Tip #94: Art Therapy

Mankind has always enjoyed and appreciated the healing power of art. The ability to express ideas and emotions visually is recognized as an effective catalyst for personal growth and development. Many consider Art Therapy a direct development of Anthroposophically Extended Medicine, but it wasn't seen as a separate profession in this country until the 1940s.

Educators have long known that children's art demonstrates their emotional and cognitive growth, but psychiatrists began using artwork created by their patients as part of their healing process early in the last century. The creative process of art can enhance recovery and contribute to health, wellness and most importantly a reduction in chronic pain.

Art therapists are professionals trained in both art and therapy. The regulation of art therapists varies by state, so please check the situation in your area when looking for an art therapist. In many areas they can become licensed as counselors or mental health therapists. The American Art Therapy Association was founded in 1969 and is the professional organization for this field while the separate Art Therapy Credentials Board certifies the education and experience of therapists.

Tip #95: Music Therapy

Although Music Therapy dates back to ancient times, the modern concept originated in veterans' hospitals after the wars when doctors noticed the beneficial physical and emotional responses of patients to music from visiting musicians. Today it improves the quality of life for children and adults suffering from chronic pain, disabilities or disease by improving motor skills, social and cognitive development and even spiritual awareness. A music therapist frequently combines Music Therapy techniques with broader types of therapy.

Patients do not have to have any musical abilities to benefit from Music Therapy. There isn't one particular type of music that is more beneficial than others. The type of music chosen for therapy will depend on the patient's preferences, situation and type of assistance needed. Listening to music you enjoy will relieve stress but hearing music you dislike can create it. Music can be used to help motor skills develop in children with special needs or adults recovering from stroke. Simply listening to music can help memory function in the elderly. Classical and jazz music are often credited with improving mental functions due to their complex arrangements.

Stress reduction is a popular form of music therapy that does not require a trained therapist. Listening to your favorite music works on many levels to wash away the stress of the day, often called a "sound bath." For best results enjoy at least twenty minutes of slow music with a rhythm of less than 72 beats per minute—the natural heartbeat. Concentrate on the silence between the notes to keep your mind from analyzing the music and remember to focus on slow, rhythmic breathing. This type of music therapy can even be combined with exercise when you take your favorite tunes on a walk.

Professional music therapists often are designated by MT-BC (Music Therapist, Board-Certified) or the designation of CMT, ACMT, or RMT. Today the American Music Therapy Association sets the standards for education and clinical training. Music Therapy may be covered by government or private insurance, so remember to check with your provider.

Tip #96: Reflexology

Reflexology is based on the concept that the nerves in the feet, hands and even our ears correspond to every part of the human body and their stimulation will increase circulation, natural healing while reducing stress, all of which is beneficial to reducing pain. If stepping on a tack can cause pain and trigger the fight-or-flight response then the same pathways can be used by reflexology to relax and heal the body.

Reflexology was discovered by three doctors in the 20th century. Dr. William Fitzgerald, an ear, nose and throat specialist, introduced his concepts in *Zone Therapy* in 1917. His process was based on the premise that the reflex areas on the feet and hands were linked to other areas of the body in the same zone. He described ten long vertical zones in the body. In 1924 Dr. Joe Shelby Riley published his book *Zone Reflex*, which added horizontal zones for the first time. Eunice Ingham, a nurse and therapist, refined the process in the 1930s into what is known today as foot reflexology and began to bring it to lay people. In 1957, French doctor, Paul Nogier, discovered the existence of an inverted reflex map of the body in the outer ear. In the early 1980s, Bill Flocco added Ear Reflexology to the field along with the concept of integrating all three types of Reflexology into the same session for maximum effectiveness.

Reflexology encourages the body to heal naturally and helps it to maintain health. Reducing stress is known to improve immune system function and increase energy levels. The process is used primarily on the feet to stimulate the flow of life energy (chi or qi). Treatments usually last for an hour but each client is unique and a course of sessions may be needed. Consistency appears to improve results but the timing will vary with each situation. Some Reflexologists recommend one session each day for six consecutive days, while others prefer once each week for six weeks or as long as needed.

As with any therapy,, if you have any questions or concerns please check with your physician. Your reflexologist may suggest a shorter session if you have certain types of health problems. Please exercise caution during the first trimester of pregnancy. For comfort and greater relaxation, you should not have a session less than one hour after meals and immediately after a session you should drink plenty of water. Reflexologists do not diagnose, prescribe or treat for specific illnesses or diseases. Always research the training and certification of a therapist.

National certification for reflexologists is done by the American Reflexology Certification Board. You can also check to be sure that your reflexologist was trained by a school accredited by the

American Commission for Accreditation of Reflexology Education and Training (see www.acaret.org). There are several how-to books and videos available for self-help along with products such as reflexology socks, which provide zone stimulation of the feet. There are also many medical research studies on the benefits of Reflexology available.

Tip #97: Tai Chi

Tai Chi is a soft style, or relaxed, form of the martial arts. It is based on the Yin/Yang concept of meeting hard with soft, using leverage rather than muscle tension to neutralize attacks. The easily recognizable slow, gentle, flowing movements of Tai Chi have been seen in large crowds across China and around the world. It is often seen as a kind of moving meditation. It follows many of the principles of Traditional Chinese Medicine and has many reported health benefits, especially for the elderly. Researchers have found the long-term Tai Chi practice has favorable effects in balance, flexibility, cardiovascular fitness with reports of reduced pain, stress and anxiety in healthy subjects. It has also been shown to decrease falls in the elderly.

There are many different styles, but they're based on the system originally taught by the Chen family to the Yang family beginning in 1820. Training involves learning the solo routines called "forms." There is also advanced training known as "pushing hands" for two people and also weapons training. There are several major styles of Tai Chi, each named after the Chinese family where it originated. These are: Chen Style; Yang Style; Wu Style; Hao Style; Sun Style and Zhaobao Style. In 1956, the Chinese Sports Committee shortened the Yang Family form to 24 postures, often called the Short Form of Tai Chi. The longer traditional solo forms can have 88 to 108 postures. In 1976, a combination form called the Combined 48 Forms was created. Today there are dozens of new styles and hybrids which have grown out of the main styles.

In 1970, Taoist Tai Chi was introduced to the West by Master Moy Lin-Shin. This form is different because it is designed to promote and restore health. The Taoist Style uses greater stretching and turning in all of the movements to increase the benefits of Tai Chi.

There is no universal certification process for Tai Chi so almost anyone can call themselves a teacher. As with all exercise programs, it is wise to first check with your physician and also carefully research the training and experience of the Tai Chi instructor.

Tip #98: Quantum Techniques

Quantum Techniques (QT) is a technique of energy medicine to identify and eliminate problems in the body's energy system that are preventing the body from healing itself. While traditional medicine tends to focus on a single cause of a disease, energy medicine works on a holistic basis. Stress, pathogens, traumas, toxins and a variety of other contributors often work together to cause disease or illness so there probably isn't going to be a single-issue solution to solve it. Treating only one facet or symptom of the problem would be ineffective. This technique is especially useful for chronic problems.

Quantum Techniques work to improve the function within the body's energy field. A person may have the correct amount of vitamins and minerals, water, proteins, carbohydrates and other elements in their body but if there is a communication failure within the body then function suffers. Each type of cell has a unique frequency. Diseased cells have different frequencies than healthy cells of the same type. Restoring the proper energy frequency removes the barriers so the body can heal itself.

The technique was developed by Dr. Stephen Daniel, a psychotherapist and then a psychologist for 22 years prior to retiring as a psychologist to work in bioenergetic medicine. Twenty-five years of daily migraines led him to develop QT, which he says "… has provided more healing in my life than any other modality." Dr. Daniel has been trained in energy processes by Dr. Roger Callahan (*look up Callahan Technique*), by Dr. Nambudripad (*see also NAET*) and is a conference presenter on the EFT series on chronic illness along with training in other energy medicine techniques.

Tip #99: Asian Bodywork

Asian Bodywork Therapy (ABT) is based upon Traditional Chinese Medicine although some forms only have roots in TCM. Treatments of the body, spirit and mind with ABT involve restoring the flow and balance of the life force or chi (chee) by manipulation and pressure.

The foundational forms of ABT are Amma, Shiatsu and Medical Qigong, but there are many different forms including: Acupressure, AMMA Therapy®, Chi Nei Tsang, Five Element Shiatsu, Integrative Eclectic Shiatsu, Japanese Shiatsu; Jin Shin Do® Bodymind Acupressure, Macrobiotic Shiatsu, Shiatsu Anma Therapy, Nuad Bo Rarn, Tuina, and Zen Shiatsu.

Amma—the traditional Korean style of bodywork based upon the Chinese form.

Anma means "push-pull" for the style of deep-tissue manipulation used along with acupressure and other points.

Chi Nei Tsang begins the energy flow in the navel area and then guides the healing power to other parts of the body.

Five Element Shiatsu relies on the traditional four cornerstones of diagnosis in TCM, which are observation, listening, asking and touch. The radial pulse is a key facet of the diagnosis since it often provides crucial information. Locating the disharmony in the body is the basis for determining the best course of treatment.

Integrative Eclectic Shiatsu combines Japanese Shiatsu with TCM and a Westernized style of soft-tissue manipulation along with dietary and herbal treatments.

Japanese Shiatsu uses finger pressure, usually the thumbs, along complete meridian lines.

Jin Shin Do® Bodymind Acupressure uses deep pressure with techniques to focus the mind and body.

Macrobiotic Shiatsu is based on the belief that every person is a part of nature. Treatment uses hand and bare foot pressure to improve the flow of chi along with dietary guides, medicinal plants, breathing techniques and corrective exercises.

Shiatsu Anma Therapy combines the energy system of TCM with modern pressure therapy.

Nuad Bo Rarn is the traditional Thai bodywork style based upon Indian Buddhist medicine and TCM along with a spiritual focus.

Tuina is a type of Chinese bodywork using soft-tissue massage along with herbal medicines and therapeutic exercises.

Zen Shiatsu—The American Organization for Bodywork Therapies of Asia (AOBTA®) is the main professional organization for this field, but the National Certification Commission for Acupuncture and Oriental Medicine (NCCAOM) provides the entry certification for ABT.

Tip #100: Myofascial Release

Myofascial Release is a technique of sustained pressure for eliminating pain and increasing the body's range of motion, which makes it perfect for dealing with chronic pain. Injuries, stress, trauma, overuse and poor posture can cause restriction to the fascia, which is just under your skin. The fascia system is a single network of coverings on muscles, bones and organs that runs from head to foot connecting every part of the body. Its normal healthy condition is relaxed, with the ability to stretch and move. When muscles are injured, stressed or inflamed, their fibers and the surrounding fascia become short and tight, a condition that can spread to other locations in the body, restricting motion and causing discomfort.

Myofascial release frees fascial restrictions and allows the muscles to move efficiently. This is usually done by applying shear, compression or tension in various directions, or by skin rolling.

Dr. Janet Travell began using the term "Myofascial Trigger Point" in 1976, so a variation of the technique is known as Myofascial Trigger Point Therapy. Practitioners using the direct method or deep tissue work use their knuckles, elbows or tools with sufficient pressure to slowly sink into the constricted fascia to stretch the fibers, allowing the tissue to reorganize into a more flexible manner.

A more gentle approach using lighter pressure is called the indirect method. This employs a stretching motion to allow the fascia to release or unwind itself. This technique uses the body's natural ability for self-correction, which often produces increased blood flow to the area and warmth. The John F. Barnes' Myofascial Release Approach seminars are one source for this type of specialized training. There are also seminars available to learn how to use this technique to treat yourself.

Tip #101: The Yuen Method

The Yuen Method™, also known as Chinese Energetic Method (CEM) is a type of full-spectrum energy healing capable of healing the source of pain whether it is physical, mental, emotional or spiritual. As a 35th generation Grandmaster of Shaolin Tai Mantis Kung-Fu, Dr. Kam Yuen developed his process by blending a lifetime study of martial arts with modern Western knowledge including physiology, anatomy and quantum physics. He is also a structural engineer and Doctor of Chiropractic who is knowledgeable in nutritional therapy and homeopathy.

The Yuen Method™ is a non-invasive healthcare process that does not require clients to change their attitudes or belief systems for it to be effective in eliminating pain. The principle of energy healing is that your body functions like a computer, and is either strong or weak on any issue. Pain is simply a warning light that there is a problem with the energy flow in the body. Practitioners use their own energy to locate the highest frequency of pain, since it is what distorts our body image and allows disease to occur.

Energetic corrections are made by the practitioner directing healing energy into the proper location and level, producing instantaneous results. The explanation for this effect is that the healing takes place at the quantum level of pure energy where everything is connected to everything else and time is not a barrier. By aligning all levels of consciousness, pain is simply eliminated.

Tip #102: Ozone or Oxygen Therapy

Ozone Therapy is a healing treatment that introduces ozone into the body. All 30 or so oxygen therapies, including ozone therapy, flood the body with single atoms (oxygen is O^2 and ozone is O^3). By putting large quantities of ozone into the body, the single oxygen molecule that is unattached circulates freely to attack a wide range of illness and disease. It is considered to be anti-viral, anti-bacterial, and anti-fungal because these organisms cannot live in an oxygen-rich environment. It is also said to have antioxidant stimulating capabilities.

This process normally uses an oxygen generator connected with an ozone generator to produce precisely controlled amounts of ozone. It may be introduced into the body in a variety of ways including:

- Ingestion: drinking water or consuming olive oil that has been infused with ozone.
- Rectal Insufflation: introducing ozone through the colon.
- Vaginal Insufflation: introducing ozone into the female body.
- Insertion in the Ear: placing the tube directly into the ear.
- Transdermal (or through the skin): using a variety of methods including a bath, body suit, wraps or bagging, and other techniques.
- Injection: placing ozone directly into the body in specially-prepared fluids, sometimes directly into a tumor site.
- Inhalation: breathing in ozone directly, often using a sauna.

In America the first use of ozone therapy was by Dr. John H. Kellogg at his Battle Creek, Michigan sanitarium using ozone steam saunas in 1880. Since that time, ozone therapy has been recognized in several countries around the world as an effective healing therapy.

The Message

After you've read all of these tips for dealing with chronic pain and yet you're still suffering, then it may be time to ask yourself "What's the message?" There are times when your subconscious mind needs to communicate an important message to your conscious mind and pain is a common way to get your attention. Finding and listening to that message may be the only way to make your pain disappear.

Wrapping all of this up, I first want to wish you the best of luck in finding a treatment, medication or therapy to help you handle your chronic pain. Regardless of the cause or causes of your pain, I hope you can get rid of it and enjoy the wonderful life you deserve.

There is growing hope for chronic pain sufferers. Clinical investigators have tested chronic pain patients and found that they often have lower-than-normal levels of endorphins in their spinal fluid. Investigations of acupuncture include wiring the needles to stimulate nerve endings electrically (electroacupuncture), which some researchers believe activates endorphin systems. Other experiments with acupuncture have shown that there are higher levels of endorphins in cerebrospinal fluid following acupuncture. Investigators are studying the effect of stress on the experience of chronic pain. Chemists are synthesizing new analgesics and discovering painkilling virtues in drugs not normally prescribed for pain.

But for now, chronic pain persists. Pain signals keep firing in the nervous system for weeks, months, even years. There may have been an initial mishap—sprained back, serious infection, or there may be an ongoing cause of pain like arthritis, cancer, ear infection, but some people suffer chronic pain in the absence of any past injury or evidence of body damage. Many chronic pain conditions affect older adults. Common chronic pain complaints include headache, low back pain, cancer pain, arthritis pain, neurogenic pain (pain resulting from damage to the peripheral nerves or to the central nervous system itself), psychogenic pain (pain not due to past disease or injury or any visible sign of damage inside or outside the nervous system). A person may have two or more coexisting chronic pain conditions, which can include chronic fatigue syndrome, endometriosis, fibromyalgia, inflammatory bowel disease, interstitial cystitis, temporomandibular joint (TMJ) dysfunction, and vulvodynia. It's not known whether these disorders share a common cause or even if that matters.

Your pain is your pain, unique and individual, it's all yours. Hopefully you'll find your answer sooner rather than later.

About The Author

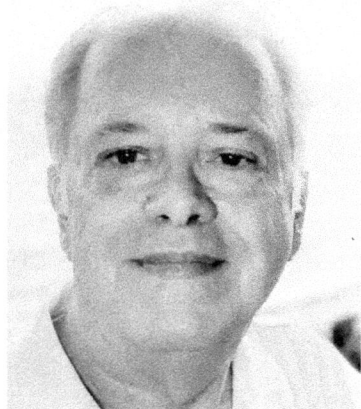

I put my journalism degree to work again doing research and interviews in 2005. My first health book was published in 2007. *How To UnBreak Your Health* received lots of very positive reviews including *Midwest Book Review, Reader Views, Clarion Reviews* and *Booksville Literary Reviews* along with many others. After a few years and more research the updated edition was published, *How To UnBreak Your Health,* which featured over 300 listings in more than 150 different categories. Once again it was published by Loving Healing Press.

A few years later I decided to try my hand at fiction so I wrote an novella, *Susan's Search.* It was about what happens when your search for a solution to your health problem takes you far from home and disrupts your life.

More recently I wrote a book on a single topic, *101 Tips for Better and More Healthy Sleep.* This shorter, more focused format seemed to be more in line with the times and what readers were looking for in a health book. It was published in 2023.

My latest book, *101 Tips for Chronic Pain Relief,* is the book I'd wish I'd written in the beginning. I've watched chronic pain can do a person's life, slowly eating away at them until the body finally gives up and dies. My mother had a new surgical procedure developed in Europe to relieve the pain in her spine many years ago. It didn't work. Nearly ten years later the pain finally ended her life, she'd just turned 40.

No one wants to suffer from chronic pain but if it happens to you, the only thing you want is for the pain to end. That's why I wrote this book, to help you find relief from your pain regardless of what it takes.

I've also recorded dozens of podcast programs on a wide variety health treatments which are still available at:
https://www.unbreakyourhealth.com/podcasts.html

Index

ABT, 106, 107
acupressure, 46, 96, 106
acupuncture defined, 55
Acupuncture, 55
Alexander Technique, 82, 83, 84
Amma, 106
Ananda yoga, 80
Anodyne Therapy, 10
Apitherapy, 100
applied kinesiology, 72, 73, 90
aromatherapy, 60, 95
Art Therapy, 101
arthrostim, 90
asanas, 79, 80
Ashtanga yoga, 80, 82
Asian Bodywork Therapy. See ABT
Ayurveda, 59, 60, 96
Ayurvedic, 60, 87
Bach Flower Remedies, 92–94
Bee-Venom Therapy. See Apitherapy
biofeedback, 65, 72 defined, 7
Birch, B.B., 82
Brahan, 81
Buddhism, 49, 50, 79, 89

Buddhist, 61, 107
CBT, 53, 54
chakras, 81, 96, 97
Chi, 87, 91
Chi Nei Tsang, 106
Chinese Energetic Method, 108
chiropractic, 72, 90
chiropractors, 62, 72
clinical hypnosis, 45
Cognitive Behavioral Therapy. See CBT
cold laser therapy, 10
colonics, 17
conscious breathing, 85
Contrology, 71
cortisol, 100
Craniosacral Therapy, 85
Crystal Bowl Therapy, 97
Crystal Healing, 97
Cupping, 55
Daniel, S., 105
doshas, 60
EFT, 46, 47, 105
Electromyography, 8
electrotherapeutic techniques, 92
Electrotherapy, 91, 92
EMDR, 52
Emoto, M., 46

endorphins, 14, 37, 43
Energy Medicine, 91
essential oils, 94, 95
fascia, 77, 107, 108
FDA, 13, 37, 58, 64, 65, 88
Feldenkrais Method®, 69, 70
Five Element Shiatsu, 106
Floatation Therapy, 99
Functional Integration, 70
gait analysis, 72
Gem Therapy, 96
Goodheart, 72
Graston Technique®, 78
Hahnemann, C.F., 58
Hatha yoga, 76, 79, 80
Healing Touch, 73
Hellerwork, 74, 75
herbs, 17, 60
Hinduism, 89
Homeopathy, 57, 58, 59
Humor Therapy, 43
hydrotherapy, 17 defined, 16
hydrothermal therapy, 16
hypnosis defined, 44

Hypnotherapy, 45
Integral yoga, 81
Integrative Eclectic
    Shiatsu, 106
Integrative Yoga
    Therapy, 81
Iyengar yoga, 81
Jaffe, C.. *See* JMT
Jaffe-Mellor
    Technique, 90
Japanese Shiatsu,
    106
Jin Shin Do, 106
Jivamukti yoga, 81
JMT, 90
Kali Ray Tri Yoga,
    81
Karuna Reiki, 89
kinesiology, 72
Kundalini yoga, 81
Kung-Fu, 108
Le Page, J., 81
Lilly, J.C., 99
lymph drainage, 10
Macrobiotic
    Shiatsu, 106
Magnetic Therapy,
    87
Magnetobiology,
    87
magnetotherapeuti
    c techniques, 92
mantra meditation,
    60
massage, 98
    defined, 78
meditation
    defined, 51
    transcendental,
    51
meridians, 13, 73
    defined, 55
Millimeter Wave
    therapy, 9
Mindfulness, 48,
    49, 50

Mindfulness Based
    Stress
    Reduction, 48
MRT, 90
muscle resistance
    testing. *See*
    MRT
muscle testing, 47,
    48, 62, 72, 73
music therapy, 60,
    102
    defined, 101
Myofascial Release,
    107, 108
Myotherapy, 75, 76
NAET, 105
Nambudripad,
    D.S., 105
Naprathy, 84
neuropeptides, 64
Nordenstrom, B.,
    91, 92
olive oil, 109
osteopathic
    manipulative
    treatment, 56
Osteopathy, 56, 57,
    85
Palmer, D.D., 62
PENS, 13
Percuntaneous
    Electrical Nerve
    Stimulation. See
    PENS
Percutaneous
    Neuromodulatio
    n Therapy. See
    PNT
Phoenix Rising
    Yoga Therapy,
    81
Pilates Method, 71,
    72
Placebo Effect, 36
PNT, 13
Power yoga, 82

Prana, 60, 87
Prayer, 45, 46
Prudden, B., 75, 76
PSYCH-K, 47
Psychological
    Kinesiology. *See*
    PSYCH-K
Psychoneuroimmu
    nology, 43
psychotherapies, 52
Qigong, 60, 61,
    106
Quantum
    Techniques, 105
Raja yoga, 79
Raku Kai Reiki, 89
Rebirthing, 85
reflexology, 103,
    104
Reflexology, 102,
    103
    defined, 103
Reiki, 88
Relaxation
    Response, 51
Restricted
    Environmental
    Stimulation
    Technique, 99
Rolfing, 76
Rosch, P.J., 91
Sahara yoga, 82
sauna, 17
SCENAR, 64
self-hypnosis, 99
Shiatsu Anma
    Therapy, 106,
    107
Singing Bowl
    Therapy, 97
Sivananda Yoga, 82
Smith, O., 84
SomatoEmotional
    Release, 86
sonupuncture, 56
Still, A.T., 56

Structural
  Integration. See
  Hellerwork
Svaroopa® yoga, 82
Tai Chi, 61, 104,
  105
Taoist, 61, 104
Tapping, 47
TCM, 55, 91, 106,
  107

TENS, 13, 64
TFT, 46
thermotherapeutic
  techniques, 92
Tibetan Yoga, 82
Transcendental
  Meditation, 51
Tuina, 106, 107
ultrasound, 84
veterinarians, 97

Viniyoga, 82
Watsu, 98
White Lotus yoga,
  82
Yin/Yang, 60, 80,
  91, 104
yoga
  defined, 79
Yuen, K., 108

ALAN E. SMITH

101

TIPS for BETTER and MORE HEALTHY SLEEP

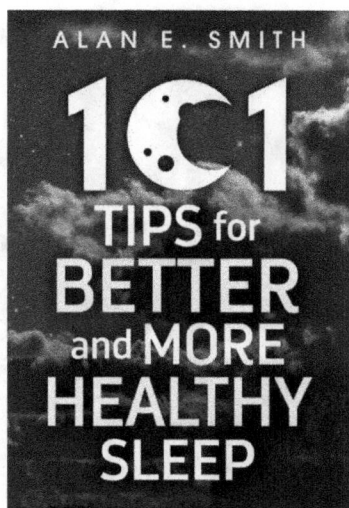

All of your physical and mental health depends on getting a good night's sleep. We all love waking up without an alarm, feeling rested and refreshed, right? Unfortunately, many people don't sleep enough or sleep well, or both. It may feel like your sleep is a combination lock and you can't figure out all the right numbers in the right sequence. These tips are designed to help you put it all together.

These *101 Tips* are designed to help you find the rest you deserve in the best way possible. You'll walk through all of the various factors in getting a good night's sleep, from your bed and bedroom to relaxing before bed to solving several sleep problems. While some of these tips have been around for hundreds or thousands of years, some are as new as they can be. We even talk about the progress that's been made in the medical field regarding sleep in past few decades.

Whatever your sleep situation, you will probably find something here that can help you sleep even better and longer. You just have to have the patience and dedication to solve your own sleep problems.

- Discover your best sleep possible
- See new ways to sleep better, longer
- Realize all of the ways to improve your sleep
- Explore techniques from ancient to modern
- Understand the real importance of sleep

Learn more at www.UnbreakYourHealth.com

Paperback * Hardcover * eBook * Audiobook

From Loving Healing Press

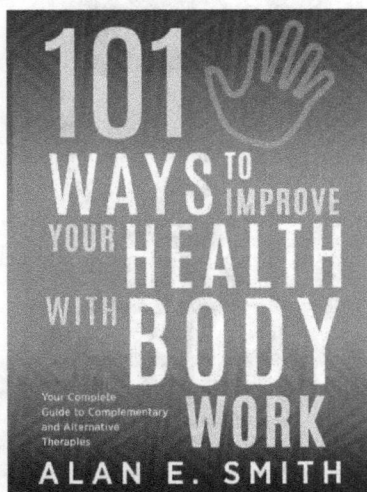

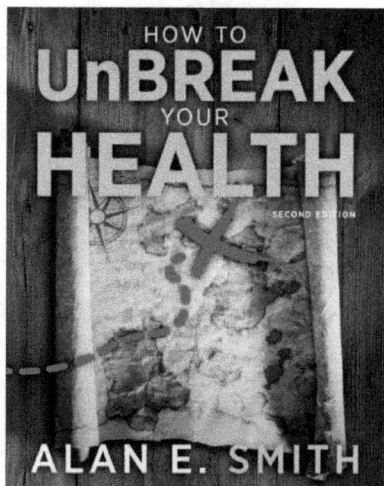

Find better health with your map to the world of complementary and alternative therapies in this comprehensive health and wellness guide for mind, body, and spirit.

Are you sinking into the Quicksand of Pain? Are you stranded in the Mountains of Misery or simply lost in a Forest of Symptoms? Find your way to Hope with the 2nd edition of the award-winning book *How To UnBreak Your Health: Your Map to the World of Complementary and Alternative Therapies*. Discover how your body, mind and energy/spirit can work together to produce better health. Learn how to take charge of your health and find your path to the best health possible.

Trying to figure out where you are with your health problems, where you need to go and the best way to get there? You need a map to find your way around the amazing world of complementary or alternative therapies! Which therapies are right for you and your health problems? Find out in this easy-to-read guide to all of the therapies available outside the drugs-and-surgery world of mainstream medicine.

- Discover health opportunities from Acupuncture to Zen Bodytherapy.

- Find out about the health benefits of Pilates, Yoga, and Massage.

- Learn about devices from Edgar Cayce's Radiac to the newest cold lasers.

- Hear from real people who've experienced these therapies and products.

- Locate free podcasts on the therapies you want to learn more about.

Kelly Bouldin Darmofal suffered a severe TBI in 1992; currently she holds a Masters in Special Education from Salem College, NC. Her memoir *Lost In My Mind: Recovering From Traumatic Brain Injury (TBI)* tells her story of tragedy and triumph. Kelly will be teaching "TBI: An Overview for Educators" at Salem College. Kelly's "tips" were learned during two decades of recovery and perseverance; they include:

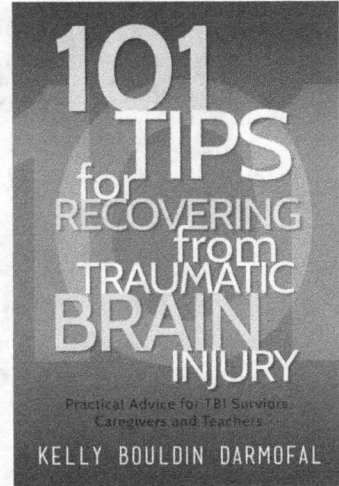

- Ways to avoid isolation and culture shock post-TBI
- Tips for staying organized in the face of instant chaos
- Strategies for caretakers and teachers of TBI survivors
- Life philosophies that reject despair
- How to relearn that shoes must match
- Why one alarm clock is never enough, and
- A breath of humor for a growing population with a "silent illness"--TBI

Those who suffer from TBI should benefit from Kelly Darmofal's advice. She speaks often of the value of a sense of humor in dealing with TBI symptoms and quotes Viktor Frankl who believed that humor was one of the "...soul's weapons in the fight for self preservation." I strongly recommend her work.
—Dr. George E. Naff, NCC, LPC, Diplomate in Logotherapy

Learn more at www.ImLostInMyMind.com

From Loving Healing Press www.LHPress.com

www.ingramcontent.com/pod-product-compliance
Lightning Source LLC
Chambersburg PA
CBHW052220270326
41931CB00011B/2421